Sneeze-Free Dog Breeds

Diane Morgan

Project Team
Editor: Heather Russell-Revesz
Copy Editor: Joann Woy
Design Concept: Leah Lococo
Design Production: Tilly Grassa

T.F.H. Publications
President/CEO: Glen S. Axelrod
Executive Vice President: Mark E. Johnson
Publisher: Christopher T. Reggio
Production Manager: Kathy Bontz

T.F.H. Publications, Inc.
One TFH Plaza
Third and Union Avenues
Neptune City, NJ 07753

Printed and bound in China
06 07 08 09 10 1 3 5 7 9 8 6 4 2

Library of Congress Cataloging-in-Publication Data
Morgan, Diane, 1947-
Sneeze-free dog breeds : allergy management and breed selection for the allergic dog lover / Diane Morgan.
  p. cm.
ISBN 0-7938-0571-6 (alk. paper)
1. Dog breeds. 2. Dogs—Selection. 3. Allergens—Control. 4. Allergy. I. Title.
SF426.M6793 2006
636.7'1—dc22
2005030536

The leader in responsible animal care for over 50 years.™
www.tfhpublications.com

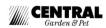

Table of Contents

Chapter 1: **Welcome to Allergy World** 5

Chapter 2: **Keep the Dog, Kick the Sneeze:**
Treatment and Management 17

Chapter 3: **Beyond the Hype in Hypoallergenic Breeds** 39

Chapter 4: **Meet the Breeds** 49

Part 1: Curly-Coated and Corded Breeds 50

Part 2: Hairless Breeds 80

Part 3: Single-Coated and Low-Shedding Breeds 98

Part 4: Terrier-Type Breeds 118

Glossary 147

Resources 151

Index 157

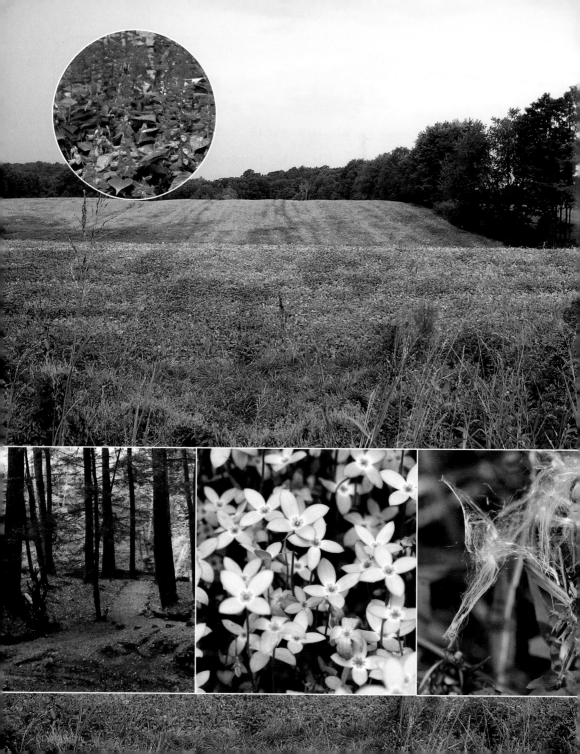

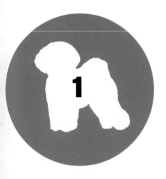

Welcome to Allergy World

THE EARTH IS A BEAUTIFUL PLANET, rich with animals, plants, and minerals. But, for millions of people, this magnificent land lurks with dangers. Every spring breeze wafts a billion particles of dust, pollen, dead skin, chemicals, and pet hair through your yard and home. Your clothes, your nose, your eyes, your skin—every receptor and covering you own is a trap for allergy-causing substances of all colors, sizes, and descriptions.

Allergies are the most widespread chronic condition in the world. More than ten million Americans (about 15 percent of the population) suffer from some sort of a pet allergy, and about 70 percent of American families own a cat or dog. With our infinite creativity, we humans have developed a number of exciting ways to respond to allergies: We sneeze. We cough. We itch. Our eyes turn red or swell shut. Our nose runs. We get sick to the stomach. We blossom with rashes. Our tonsils swell. We stop breathing.

Well, it makes sense (at least sort of) to be allergic to poison ivy, ragweed, or MSG. But allergic to the family pet? It seems so unfair, especially when you consider that an allergy may appear literally overnight (although it may have been months or years in the making).

> People who have asthma are at increased risk for pet allergies as well.

It's a popular belief that animal hair causes allergies but, with pets, the villainous substance is *not* hair. Allergies are triggered by special proteins called *allergens* (even though hair is made of protein, it's not the same kind) secreted by oil glands and shed with dan-

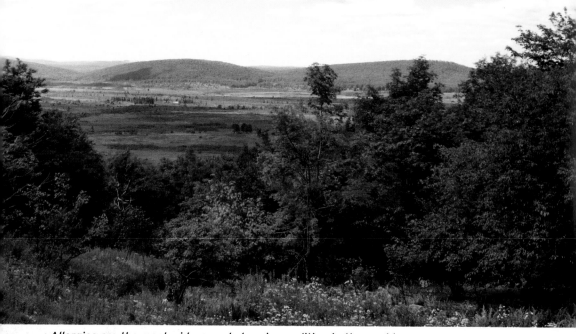

Allergies are the most widespread chronic condition in the world.

der. (In an example of lexical redundancy, allergens are those substances that trigger an allergic reaction.) Allergenic proteins are abundant in the saliva, which indeed clings to hair when a dog licks itself. Still more allergens can be found in the urine.

The good news is that allergies can be controlled, if not beaten. The days are gone when allergies could keep you from what you most love—whether it's the world outside, a dusty library, or your beloved Fido.

CATS VERSUS DOGS

Dog allergies are about half as frequent as cat allergies–four out of five people who are allergic to animals are allergic to cats. Some suggest this is because cats lick themselves so much. Because cats are more likely to cause allergic reactions than are dogs, most of the research on pet allergies has been done on them.

Cat allergens have been detected in homes for months after the departure of the cat, and have even been discovered in the Antarctic, although no cats have ever been there! Researchers have learned that longer-haired cats tend to shed fewer allergens. It is not currently known if this is true for dogs.

Some people who are allergic to their own pets have no severe or immediate increase of their symptoms when they are near their them. Instead, they suffer from continual low-grade symptoms that clear up only after days or even weeks away from the house.

IS IT OVER FOR ROVER?

The days are also gone when doctors automatically advised their patients to "get rid of the dog." More responsive practitioners understand that's not even an option for many who already own and love their pets, or even for those who have dreamed of dog owner-ship all their lives. Some people (like farmers) depend on animals for their livelihood, while still others can benefit from the assistance of a guide or helper dog.

Getting rid of animals is not even practi-cal. Researchers at the National Institute for Environmental Health Sciences (NIEHS) discov-ered that pet allergens were present in every single one of the 831 homes tested across the United States. *This included homes of non–pet owners.* Nine percent of the homes without a dog had high enough levels of allergen to cause asthma symptoms in asthmatics who were allergic to dogs. The suggested explana-tion is that dog and cat proteins are "sticky," clinging to clothes and shoes. So, even if you find the dog another home, his allergens will remain. (The vacuum samples from the study showed that couches had the highest concen-trations of allergens, even in petless homes,

suggesting that residents or visitors brought the allergen material in on their clothing and then plopped down on the couch.)

This means these same sticky proteins are everywhere—movie theater seats, clothing

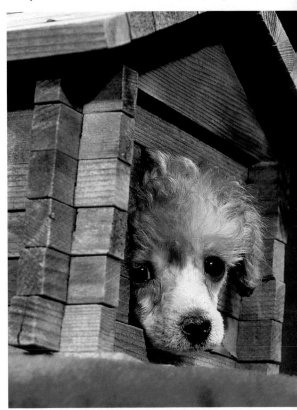

Gone are the days when doctors automatically advised their patients to "get rid of the dog."

stores, airplane and train seats, even your allergist's office! (For more details, check out the NIEHS website at www.niehs.nih.gov/oc/news/dogcata.htm.)

This study also suggests that "getting rid of the dog" won't solve the problem for these allergy sufferers. It is agonizing for families to have to remove a beloved pet, especially if several children are present in a household and only one is allergic. And, in fact, most pet owners (between 75 and 90 percent) do not "get rid of the dog." They learn to live with it, and you can too. You can fight back, and you can win the allergy battle.

Part of the fight is finding an allergist who will help you in your battle against pet dander without insisting you "get rid" of the pet. Not every allergist is so enlightened.

Before we talk about what breed of dog might be best for you, let's explore a little bit about what allergies are, and what causes them.

WHAT IS AN ALLERGY?

An allergy, in simplest terms, is part of the immune system gone wacky. Now, the immune system is a very good thing, when it's working properly. It protects us from bacteria, viruses, and lots of nasty things we come in contact with. But the immune system can go bad, just like other body systems can. For most allergy

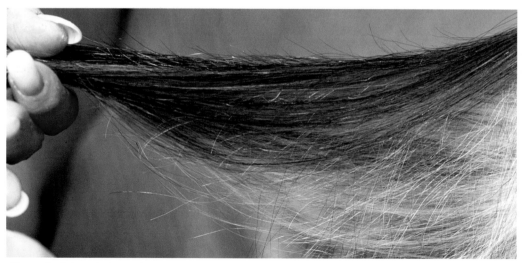

The culprit is not dog hair, but the dander clinging to the hair.

sufferers, the immune system is just slightly miscalibrated. For others, it can turn deadly.

An allergy is really a false alarm of the immune system, a situation in which the immune system is tricked into thinking that a harmless particle of pet dander is an invading army of deadly pathogens. This is one reason why allergies are called "hypersensitivity" reactions (and they're not referring to your emotions).

Immunology 101

While immunology is a difficult and arcane branch of medical science, the basics are simple enough. The culprits of allergies are antibodies in the bloodstream. The particular antibody we are concerned with here is *immunoglobulin E* (IgE), a substance discovered in the 1960s, the so-called "allergy antibody." It's the one that causes those acute, immediate allergic reactions.

Immunoglobulins are a kind of large-molecule protein, shaped like the letter Y. The body's immune system can tailor the immunoglobin molecules to precisely fit the shape of the allergen. When the allergen comes in contact with the immunoglobin, the antibody is "turned on," like a key in a lock. It goes into action, and you suffer the allergy symptoms.

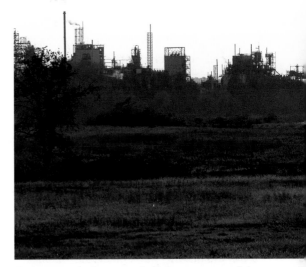

Process emissions can irritate some people's allergies.

Nobody is sure what the original purpose of IgE was—some experts think it was intended to deal with internal parasites. (Apparently it's good stuff to have around if you're living in the jungle and likely to get river blindness or schistosomiasis. Ugh.) In contemporary industrialized countries however, the stuff seems to do more harm than good. But we're stuck with it.

Apparently bored with not having enough parasites to fight, IgE gloms onto *mast cells* (special cells found in the mucosal tissue of the lungs, skin, tongue, and the linings of the nose and intestinal tract) and

Immunoglobulin and antibody mean approximately the same thing.

basophils (a special kind of white blood cell). Both basophils and mast cells are *granulocytes* that contain powerful "granules" loaded with potent chemicals that allow the cells to destroy foreign bodies. One of these powerful chemicals is *histamine*, which is responsible for allergies and inflammation as well as immunity. When the histamine is released onto the *receptor cells,* those cells undergo biochemical changes and produce the familiar symptoms of allergies: the nose starts to run...You get the picture.

IgE in the Blood

When we are born, the level of IgE circulating in the bloodstream is very low compared to other immunoglobulins. In fact, it's almost nonexistent (although some studies

---

ANTIBODY FACTS

- Histamines are the most famous, but not the only, chemicals released by the IgE-mast cell combo. Others include certain prostaglandins, bradykinin, and something called substance P.
- Humans make four other kinds of antibodies too: IgA, IgD, IgG, and IgM. But you can forget about them—thankfully, they're irrelevant to our present purpose.

---

show that higher than normal levels in umbilical cord blood and an infant's serum predict the early onset of allergies). In adults, the more IgE present in the system, the more likely it is that the person has one or more allergies. These allergies can be expressed in many ways—allergic rhinitis (runny nose and sneezing), extrinsic asthma (breathing difficulties), atopic eczema, hives, urticaria (skin rashes), and pruritus (itching). Also, these kinds of allergies are largely inherited. A person with one allergic parent has a risk of almost 50 percent of developing an allergy him or herself. Someone with two allergic parents has a risk of 70 percent.

Sometimes the term *atopic allergy* is used to refer to the IgE-mediated (and often inherited) allergies, such as the one we are talking about here—the one to animal dander. Oddly, though, a person with an atopic disease is not at higher risk for developing an allergic reaction to an injected allergen, like a drug or a bee sting.

The Allergy Bomb

People with pet allergies aren't allergic to the cat or dog per se, but to the old skin cells (dander) that are continuously shed, and to saliva and discharge from the sebaceous glands. But dander gets the blame because dander goes airborne (and may have saliva or oil molecules on it). It's when the stuff goes

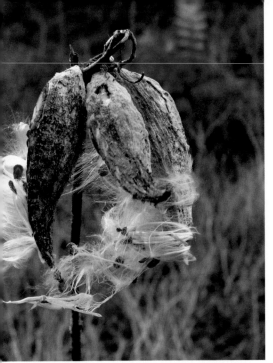

Some allergists refer to histamine as an "allergy bomb."

airborne that the problem arises.

The body can produce different kinds of IgE for different substances, thus setting off multiple allergies.

Here's what happens: You're walking innocently along. And suddenly you're exposed to, say, ragweed. The body produces IgE antibodies specific to ragweed. The interaction between the allergens and the allergen-specific IgE stimulates the cells to release histamines and other substances that affect the blood vessels, which begin the allergic reaction. Some allergists refer to histamine as an "allergy bomb."

Some allergic reactions are quite mild, maybe a little sneezing or a runny nose. In a few people, however, an allergic reaction can be extreme or even life threatening. The person cannot breathe, the heart malfunctions, and the blood pressure dives. This condition is called *anaphylaxis* and usually only occurs after an allergen injection, such as a bee sting. If you are *this* allergic to animal dander (it's practically an impossibility, since animal dander is not usually injected), you're really better off without a dog. Even a Basset Hound is not worth dying for.

IgE Facts

- IgE accounts for only about 0.001 percent of the antibody in the blood. For such a tiny amount of substance, it can certainly cause a great deal of misery.
- There's actually a disease called the Job-Buckley syndrome, in which a person has a superload of IgE, often stemming from repeated Staphylococcus bacterial infections. The person suffers weak bones and recurrent fractures as well as allergic-like symptoms.
- There's a tendency for IgE allergies to run in families, so stop blaming the dog. It's our parents' fault.
- Reagin is an old allergist's term for IgE antibodies.

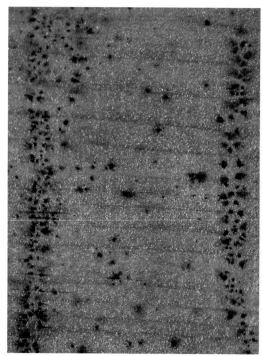
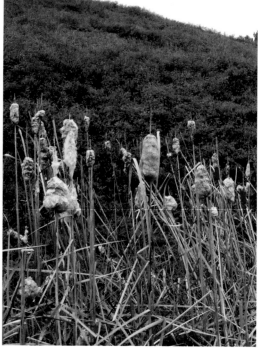

Don't just assume it's the dog! Mold, pollen or dust could be the allergy culprit.

First Exposure

Interestingly, the first exposure to an allergen doesn't result in symptoms, even for those folks who later develop an allergy. The first exposure simply encourages antibodies to be produced. With repeated exposure over a period of weeks to years, more and more histamine is released.

One great word from the allergy world is "scurf"–skin squames (scales) shed from the surface of the skin (also saliva, tears, and urine)

FINDING THE CULPRIT

The first step in handling an allergy is discovering exactly what you are allergic to. Don't just assume it's the Pomeranian—get tested. There are billions of things you might be allergic to, and the dog is only one of them. Many times the pet gets the blame, when the real culprit is dust, mold, or pollen.

Several kinds of blood tests are available to your doctor that confirm that an

Dog allergies are cumulative and may build up over time. There is a greater tendency for them to start in childhood, however, because a child's immune system is much more sensitive than that of an adult.

allergy is in fact present, but skin tests are most useful for identifying particular allergens. (In cases where a skin test can't be done, the doctor can perform a radioallergosorbent [RAST] assay, which is equally accurate, although it is more expensive and doesn't yield results as quickly).

To perform the test, the doctor will take very dilute solutions of various suspected allergens, including pollens, dust, grasses, and, of course, animal dander. They are injected individually into various parts of the skin. If you're allergic to animal dander, a red swelling will form at the site within 20 minutes. Then you know.

ALLERGIES TO ANIMAL DANDER (AND MORE)

All warm-blooded pets, regardless of hair length, produce dander, which is simply dead skin cells. These particular allergens are very, very small—approximately 2.5 microns (1 micron = 1/25,000 inch). Animal dander is extremely lightweight and can stay airborne for hours.

It's also a very sticky allergen, clinging to everything. Sebaceous (oil producing) glands in the skin also produce these protein allergens. Scientists have found that male cats

produce more of these sebaceous secretions than females (it's a function of testosterone), and there is no reason to suppose that the same isn't true of dogs. Because most dogs do not self-clean the way cats do, dogs tend to have more dander; however, it is the production of the sebaceous glands that greatly increases allergic responses.

Most symptoms develop when airborne dander comes into contact with the mucous membranes of the eyes and nose. (Animal dander can also be inhaled into the bronchial tubes.)

OTHER ALLERGENS

It's not always the dog. Guinea pigs and gerbils have strong allergens in their dander and urine. Laboratory workers, zoo personnel, and veterinarians may turn out to be allergic to lions, tigers, and monkeys.

People with mold allergy can have allergy symptoms from bird droppings and an accumulation of mold in the cage (dust can also be a problem). Fish tanks can cause symptoms because of mold growth.

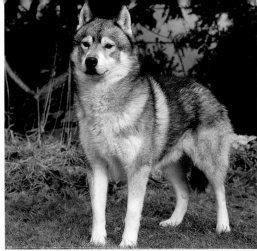
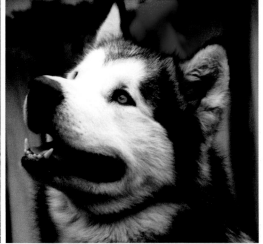
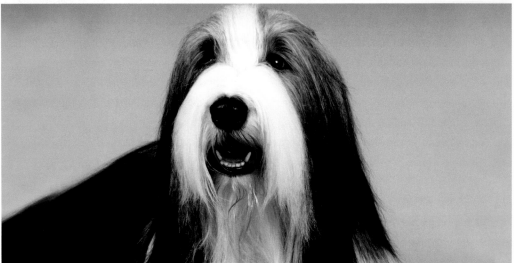

Siberian Huskies and Alaskan Malamutes "blow their coat" twice a year; Bearded Collies go through "the big shed."

Animal dander causes the particular type of allergic reaction called *perennial allergic rhinitis* (sneezing and runny nose) and comes from breathing in airborne particles of the offending dander. Most people suffering this type of allergy don't get eye inflammation, but nasal congestion that may block the Eustachian tubes in the ears and cause hearing problems, especially in kids. Complications of pet allergy can include chronic sinus headaches and infections, and asthma. It's not always easy, by the way, to tell the difference

CAT ALLERGEN

The cat allergen, invisible to the eye, is called Fel D1. This substance, deposited on the skin and coat, is more abundant in intact male cats than in females. The highest concentrations are deposited most heavily in the genital area and at the base of the tail, but since cats clean themselves so frequently, they spread it around their entire body. This allergen is particularly potent and airborne, and it can trigger an allergic reaction within minutes. The dog allergen is known as Can f1.

not growing, but thankfully, not falling out, either. In the third, or *telegen* phase, the new hair grows in, and the old hair falls out. Some breeds, like Siberian Huskies and Alaskan Malamutes, "blow their coat" twice a year, a process that takes from 3 to 6 weeks. During that time, the hair comes out in clumps (some sometimes really big clumps) and, during periods of dry heat, it gets worse.

Other breeds, like Bearded Collies, go through something called "the big shed" when they lose all their baby fur and grow in the adult kind. It's pretty hard on allergy sufferers. Other factors that can influence growth or shed are hormonal factors, heat, stress, illness, and nutritional factors.

between perennial allergic rhinitis and recurring sinus infections or growths (polyps) inside the nose. And, someone could have all three at the same time!

Dog allergies may not show up right away; in fact, they can take two or more years to develop. Most people allergic to dogs are also allergic to other things.

THE GLORY OF HAIR

Hair growth progresses naturally through a three-phase cycle. During the first phase, the *anagen* phase, the hair grows actively. When it has reached its genetically predetermined length, it stops growing. This is the second, or *catagen* phase. It just stays there,

DON'T FORGET

- Allergens are everywhere on the planet. You can't avoid them!
- An allergy is just an overstimulated or hypersensitive immune system.
- Allergies can be expressed in many different ways, but most people allergic to dogs start sneezing.
- People with allergic parents are much more likely to develop allergies themselves.
- For people with allergies to dogs, the villain is animal dander.
- While allergies can't be "cured," they can usually be controlled, even if you have a dog.

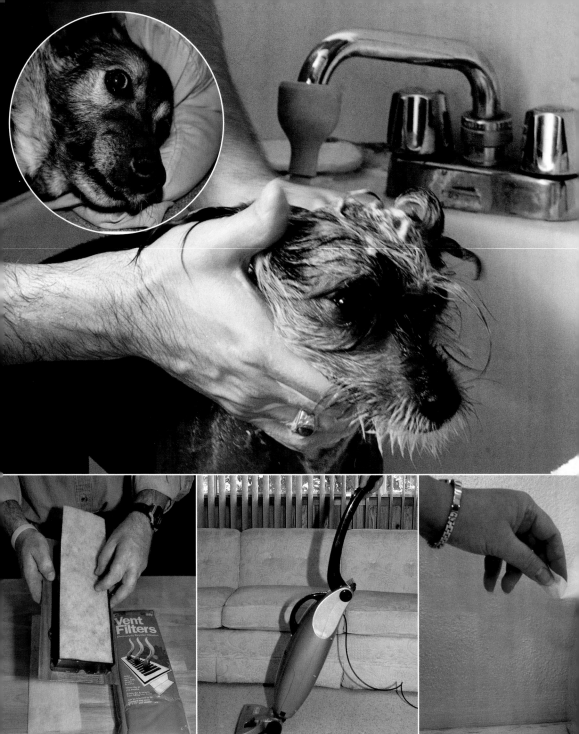

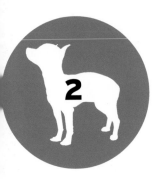

Keep the Dog, Kick the Sneeze:
Treatment and Management

DOG ALLERGIES CAN BE CONTROLLED. Unless you are one of the extremely rare people (almost nonexistent) who suffer anaphylactic reactions to dogs, you can keep your dog while you control your allergy. And by keeping the dog, I don't mean tying him out in the backyard 24 hours a day while you try to breathe. I mean keeping him *with* you.

Allergies are cumulative, and most people who are allergic to one substance are also allergic to others, such as dust, dust mites, feathers, mildew, mold, paint, perfume, pesticides, smoke, and soaps. In fact, many people allergic to dogs are so minimally allergic that the allergy manifests itself only when they are exposed to other allergens at the same time! That is, the exposure to other allergens exceeds the sufferer's "threshold level." Minimizing your exposure to other allergens may allow you keep your dog!

So, avoid other possible allergens wherever possible. Since allergic reactions are cumulative, if you are allergic to other things besides dog dander, exposure to multiple allergens vastly increases your chances of an allergy flare-up.

TREAT YOURSELF

Since you are the one with the defective (okay, hypersensitive sounds better) immune system, it only makes sense that you should start working on yourself. After all, the allergen will always be around, even if you don't own a dog.

Allergen Immunotherapy

Allergen immunotherapy is a fancy way of saying "shots." Believe it or not, allergy shots have been around since 1911, and have been greatly improved over

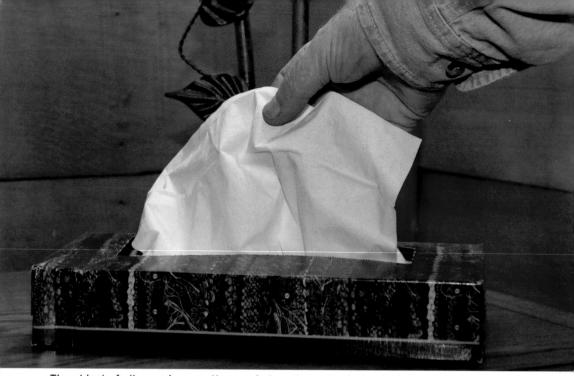

The object of allergen immunotherapy is to get your body to produce "blocking antibodies" that will prevent an allergic response, and stop you reaching for the tissue box.

the years. In this approach, tiny bits of the allergen are injected just under the skin in gradually increasing amounts until you reach "maintenance level." The maintenance injections are usually given once a week, at least at first. Later, they can be tapered off to once every 4 to 6 weeks. Your doctor will probably ask you to hang around the office for 20 min-utes or so afterwards, to make sure you don't have a reaction to the shot. If you have a mild reaction, the doctor can administer an antihistamine like diphenhydramine to block the symptoms. A severe reaction requires an injection of epinephrine.

The object of the treatment is to get your body to produce "blocking antibodies" that

Additional information on asthma and other allergic diseases is available by calling the American College of Allergy, Asthma, and Immunology (ACAAI) toll free number at (800) 842-7777 or visiting its web site at www.acaai.org.

If you or your children are allergic to dogs, but can't bear the idea of living without one, explore going for desensitizing shots before the arrival of the pet.

will prevent an allergic response. After time, the blood level of IgE antibodies will also be reduced. This is tricky therapy, however, and must be carried out under the guidance of an allergist. If too much of the allergen is injected too soon, an allergic reaction will develop. However, some people are candidates for so-called "rush" immunotherapy, a treatment regimen that speeds up the immunity-building process by introducing the increasingly larger doses of extract through several injections given over a period of 2 to 3 days. For those who can't avoid an allergen, this treatment can bring relief quickly.

While immunotherapy isn't for everyone, studies show that people with animal dander allergies are among those who respond favorably, although perhaps not quite as well as those allergic to pollen or dust mites. (In addition, it seems to work better for those with cat allergies than with dog allergies.) Treatment takes from 3 to 6 months to reach full effectiveness, and works in 60 to 80 percent of the cases. It is true, however, that cat and dog allergen immunotherapy seems to

work more effectively for those who have only occasional, unavoidable exposure, than for pet owners.

And, there's good news for those who choose this type of treatment—it may not be forever. As the injections take effect and immunity is developed, the injections can be tapered off. For many people, they can be discontinued eventually. Recent research reveals that, once immunity is developed, patients continue to experience the immunity benefits for 8 or more years after the shots have been discontinued.

Histamine blockers were first developed in 1937.

Antihistamine Treatment

Histamines are the villains in many allergic responses. They make your eyes red, your skin itch, and your nose run (not a pretty combination). If histamines are the culprits, antihistamines are part of the answer.

You body has two kinds of histamine receptors: H1 and H2. When we use the term antihistamine, though, we're talking about drugs that block the H1 receptor. (The H2 receptor blockers are used to treat peptic ulcers and heartburn.) Antihistamines relieve runny noses and eyes as well as sneezing and other minor allergy symptoms.

Tablets

Antihistamine tablets are available without a prescription and come in a variety of forms, including short-acting and extended-release. Some prescription antihistamines that are good for allergies include the following (I am listing the active generic ingredient; the brand name follows in parentheses) The asterisked substances are "non-drowsy."

- Azatadine
- Cetirizine*
- Cyproheptadine
- Dexchlorpheniramine
- Loratadine* (Claritin)
- Methdilazine
- Promethazine
- Trimeprazine
- Tripelennamine

Nonprescription antihistamines good for allergies include:

- Brompheniramine
- Chlorpheniramine (Chlor-Trimeton)
- Clemastine (Tavist)
- Dexbrompheniramine
- Diphenhydramine (Benadryl)
- Pyrilamine
- Triprolidine

In most cases, the over-the-counter stuff works as well and is much cheaper than the prescription variety. The downside of antihistamines is that many cause drowsiness. However, a few of the newer prescription brands (starred) do not cause drowsiness, because they do not penetrate the blood–brain barrier and, if sleepiness is a problem for you with most antihistamines, they might be worth inquiring about. Less frequent side effects (found mostly in older people) may include confusion, constipation, blurred vision and, in older men, problems urinating. If you have high blood

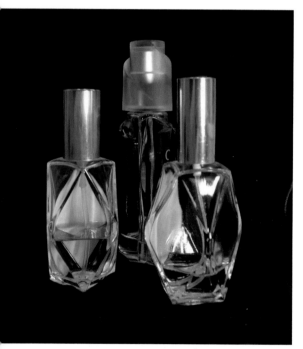

Avoid using perfumes and air fresheners in the house.

pressure, over-the-counter antihistamines can be dangerous. They raise blood pressure and can lead to a heart attack or stroke. Since antihistamines are metabolized in the liver, people with liver disease should not take them.

Often, antihistamines are the first treatment for an allergic reaction, although sometime a nasal decongestant is also used, since antihistamines don't work well for congestion or tearing eyes. But be careful—don't use a nonprescription nasal decongestant for more than a few days. They are really designed just to help people with colds, and are not for permanent allergy sufferers. After a few days of using them you may get a "rebound effect," and your nose may become even more congested than before.

New asthma medications called leukotriene modifiers (Singulair, Accolate, and Zyflo [zileuton]) can also help some people. Singulair can be prescribed for children as young as 2 years.

Eye Drops

Red, itchy eyes are a common reaction to allergens. Eye drops like Patanol, Alocril, and Zaditor help with eye tearing. Patanol starts working in about 10 minutes and lasts for 12 hours. Alocril and Zaditor need to be taken well in advance and may take a week or so to become effective.

Nasal Sprays

Prescription corticosteroid nasal sprays are very helpful, and the new ones on the market have almost no bad side effects. Nasonex is a brand that is safe for children, too. A noncorticosteroid prescription spray that sometimes works is cromolyn (pronounced CRO-moh-lin), a cromolyn-sodium nasal spray that prevents the release of histamines after contact with an allergen. Cromolyn may be used alone or with other asthma medicines, such as bronchodilators (medicines that open up narrowed breathing passages) or corticosteroids (cortisone-like medicines). An ophthalmic solution of this medicine also is available for eye problems caused by allergies. Cromolyn is sold under the name Intal.

However, some nasal sprays do make you drowsy, and others have a bitter taste. Two popular sprays without these effects are Atrovent and NasalCrom.

> To help stop tearing eyes, wet a washcloth with cold water and place over your eyes for 15 to 20 minutes.

Anti-IgE: A New (Experimental) Hope

It's a mouthful, but the anti-IgE antibody, also called rhuMAb-E25 and omalizumab (Xolair), is a recombinant humanized mono-clonal antibody to immunoglobulin E (IgE) developed to interfere early in the allergic process by targeting the source of allergy symptoms. It is very useful for patients with asthma. By binding to circulating IgE in the blood, this antibody keeps IgE from binding to the mast cells and basophils, thus blocking the release of its inflammatory chemicals. This early blockage is a departure from previous approaches that focus on symptom relief only.

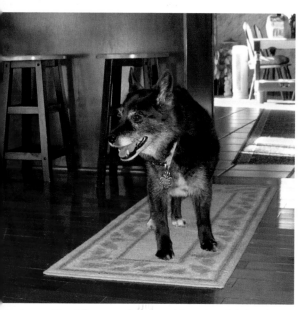

Hard floor surfaces and keeping fabrics to a minimum can help control allergens in the house.

However, omalizumab does not bind to IgE already bound to effector cells. The anti-IgE antibody is designed to be administered by injection every 2 to 4 weeks.

TREAT THE HOUSE

Your home is your castle and, to keep it that way, you need to reduce the allergens that tend to linger there. You'll also need to avoid coming in contact with as many allergens as you can, so if possible, have a nonallergic person handle cleaning chores. What a great way to get out of housecleaning duties!

The "rhu" in rhuMAb-E25 stands for "recombinant human," meaning that is a genuine human protein made in specially modified bacterial or other nonhuman cells.

See, there are some advantages to having an allergy....

Dander-Catchers Out the Door

The Bed

Allergic patients should not use feather pillows or down comforters. You can use any number of synthetic fills for pillows. One company makes a pillow called Purest Gold that is actually washable and has antimicrobial protection. If you can't live without feathers or down, encase it in plastic or an encasing with a zipper, so none of the feathers can escape. Pristine 100 microfiber is an excellent pillow cover.

Cover your mattress with a vinyl cover and change all bedding (including blankets and quilts) at least once a week. Wash your bedding in an anti-allergy detergent like Demite.

Carpets

There are no carpets in my house, and I can't think of an easier way to keep your home clean and mostly free of dander. Carpets trap dust, dander, and other allergens that are very hard to remove no matter how much you

vacuum. The allergen particles are so small they filter through the carpet and get right into the pad. Next to the pet himself, the carpet is the biggest reservoir of animal dander in the house. The more carpeted surface you have, the more dander you have (well, not

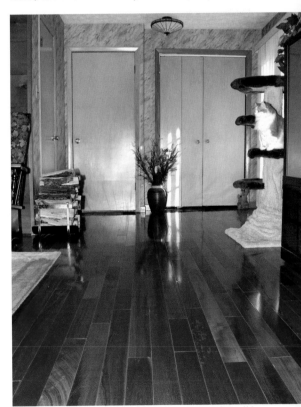

Hardwood floors are a better choice than carpet.

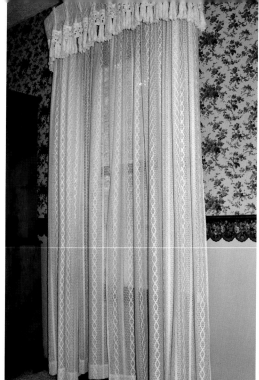
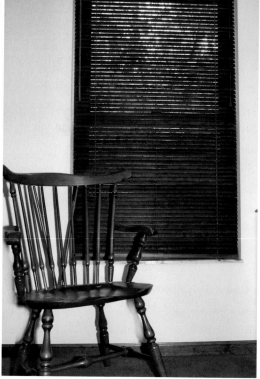

Replace old-fashioned dust-catching curtains with snazzy blinds.

you personally, of course—your house).

Hardwood floors, ceramic or vinyl tiles, and linoleum are better choices than carpets. If you absolutely must have carpets, buy one that is coated with Teflon. If you have wall-to-wall carpeting, steam clean frequently, at least every 3 months. When washing carpets or rugs, you can use a special product like Allersearch X-Mite Carpet Solution that neutralizes dust mite and other allergens and

Since pets stir up dust, having dogs and cats may also aggravate dust mite allergies in people at risk to them.

cleans both carpeted and upholstered surfaces. The rug shampoo deactivates allergens created by house dust mites, household pets, cat dander, and some kinds of pollen while cleaning and refreshing velvet, velour, corduroy, carpets, and all other pile fabrics.

Curtains and Furniture

Replace old-fashioned dust-catching curtains with snazzy vertical blinds. If you have curtains, get the kind that can come down easily, so that you can wash them every month. Even walls collect allergens, so use a long-handled brush and go over them every couple of weeks. If possible, get rid of uphol-stered furniture and replace it with a noncloth alternative, like leather or wood.

Install Air Filters and Cleaners

Air currents from forced-air heating and air-conditioning spread the allergens through-out the house, but you can fit the system with a central air cleaner. Invest in a high-efficiency particu-late air (HEPA) filter or electronic cleaner in every room of the house or in the central air–heating sys-tem to remove airborne allergens. (You can also add one to your air condi-tioning.)

This may remove sig-nificant amounts of pet allergens from the home. The air cleaner should be used at least 4 hours per day. Remember that air cleaners are good only for airborne particles, not those that have accumulat-

ed on furniture and the like. While these appliances remove most airborne particles, the benefits of a HEPA filter may be limited if there is a large reservoir of dander in furniture and carpet.

Selecting an Air Filter or Cleaner

Factors to consider when selecting a model include the size of the space in which the air filtration unit will be placed, the num-ber of times per hour the air will be complete-

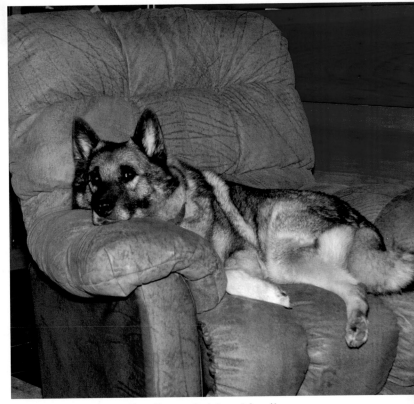

Leather is a better option than upholstered furniture.

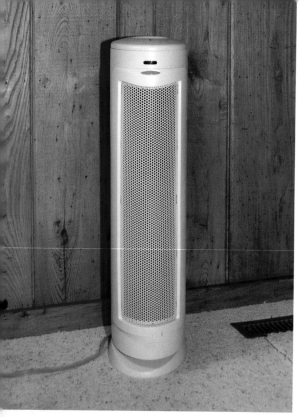
Use a room air purifier to remove airborne animal dander.

ones include Taskmaster, Panasonic, Delonghi, Lightning Air, IQAir, Blueair, CARE 2000, Honeywell Air Cleaner, Austin Air HEPA Air Cleaners, Bionair Air Cleaners, and Surround Air. Be sure that the exhaust from the air cleaner is not directed towards carpets or soft furnishings, so as not to disturb allergens that may have settled there.

Air Ducts and Air Conditioners

You should also use a filter on the air ducts in your home. Use a good-quality pleated electrostatic type, and change it every month. These prevent the spread of dust, mold spores, and dander through the duct-system point of entry. The Vent-ProHeating Vent Filter is a good choice; replace it every two months. Some people find the permanent, washable electrostatic models even more effective.

ly cycled, and the size of the particles the system will handle (the smaller the better). After all, animal dander is a mere 2.5 microns (1 micron = 1/25,000 inch). Remember to change the filters frequently. Two good brands are Taskmaster Healthmate or Pleat-A-Static high-performance allergy-free electrostatic air filters. A good inexpensive choice is the 3M Disposable Electrostatic Central Furnace Filter.

Use a room air purifier in the bedroom to remove airborne animal dander. Some good

ALLERGY TIPS

- **Always wash your hands after petting the dog, or after handling his bedding and toys.**
- **Avoid perfumed air fresheners and cleaners that can cause allergic reactions.**
- **Roughly textured fabrics hold the most allergens.**

Naturally, no one is a smoker in your home. Smoking makes everything worse for allergy sufferers!

Select the "Circulate" setting for home and car air conditioning systems to avoid introducing animal dander allergens from outside. Avoid ceiling fans—they just stir up the dander.

Window air conditioners can help with allergies, but keep them off when no one is home. Once it is turned on, stay out of the room for half an hour if you are allergic to mold; some window units emit short bursts of mold when they are first activated. Clean window air-conditioning units and humidifiers frequently to eliminate mold and mildew growth.

Lower the Humidity

Keep the humidity in your home below 45%. To measure the humidity level, you can buy an inexpensive hygrometer, available at many hardware or discount stores.

No Irritants Inside

Avoid using aerosols, sprays, paints, insecticides, chemicals, epoxy, and heavy air fresheners in the house. And, of course, ban smoking in the home. These irritants trigger allergy symptoms and compound the effects of allergens such as pet dander, dust mites, and pollen.

Open the Windows (Maybe)

Just opening the windows on a breezy day will help clean your home of dander. Or, use a fan to help push air out the window. However, if you are allergic to pollens (April through May), grasses (June through July), or ragweed (August through October) as well as pet dander, closed windows are your only option. (There is no ragweed out West, so Californians are safe.) If you have tree allergies (maple, ash, oak, elm, birch, and cedar are the most common), you'll also want to keep your windows shut.

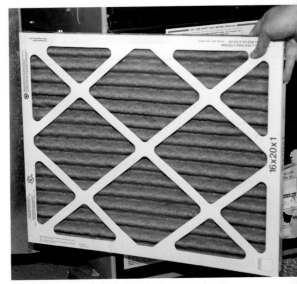

You should use a filter on the air ducts in your home.

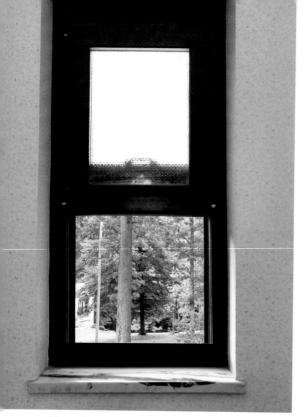

If you are allergic to pollens, grasses, ragweed, or trees opening your windows can exacerbate your allergies.

Protect Your Car

Dogs leave their dander in your car. If you travel with your pet (taking him to the vet for example), put a washable covering over the seat that will collect the dander. Then throw the cover in the wash when you return home.

Stock Up the Closet

One way to make your cleaning chores a bit easier is to stock a closet full of all your grooming and cleaning supplies. It makes it a lot easier than having everything scattered all over the house.

Try Anti-Dander Products

Several companies produce excellent anti-dander products like Allerpet, a spray you can use on your home and even on the dog or cat! Various sorts of disposable wipes developed by pet product companies provide a quick and easy way to remove loose fur from furniture (or even from the dog).

The Vacuum

Invest in a new vacuum cleaner, one with a high allergen-containment rating. Regular vacuum cleaners may actually do more harm than good, since ordinary vacuums usually don't get deep enough and may instead stir up dander. Try a HEPA vacuum filter (or double filter). Change the vacuum bags frequently—don't wait until they are full. The Panasonic vacuum clean-

---

ALLERGY SEASONS

Here are some of the most common allergens and the months when they are at their height.

- **Pollens: April through May**
- **Grasses: June through July**
- **Ragweed: August through October**

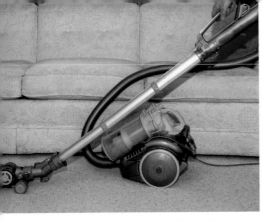

Invest in a vacuum cleaner with a high allergen-containment rating.

er with a high-efficiency HEPA filter and a Micro-lined Vacuum Bag to trap animal dander is a good choice. Run the furnace or central air conditioning fan continuously for at least 2 hours after vacuuming. Follow the vacuuming with a spray such as Allersearch ADS Anti-Allergen Dust Spray to denature the remaining allergens.

Wipe It Away

You can buy a magnetic wiping fabric that can be used on wood, metal, glass, plastic, ceramic, and on television or computer monitor screens. The magnetic fabric picks up more dander and dust than a cotton rag. To use it, just wipe lightly. Wash the fabric with a mild detergent when done. Taskmaster makes a good one.

TREAT THE DOG: DON'T GET HIS DANDER UP!

One of the best ways to keep yourself from suffering allergic symptoms is to take excellent care of your dog. Anything that injures or irritates the skin can result in the production of more dander. As an allergy sufferer, you will know that something may be wrong with your dog if you start sneezing more!

Careful grooming is the first step. This doesn't mean you have to do it—get your spouse, friend, child, or professional groomer to groom your dog, so that you can avoid excessive contact with the dander.

DRESS UP YOUR DOG!

Sweaters and other doggie apparel helps control the release of dander and control shedding. Wash the dog clothes frequently.

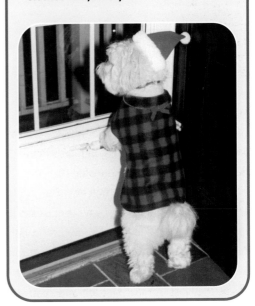

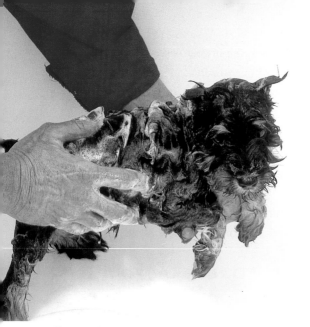

Frequent, thorough bathing is an excellent way to remove dead hair and dander from your dog.

Bathing

Frequent, thorough bathing is an excellent way to remove dead hair and dander from your dog. Research has shown that washing a pet two to three times a week can remove up to 84 percent of the surface allergen and significantly reduce the amount of future allergen produced. Unbathed animals can get irritated skin that simply makes them want to lick more and spread saliva all over their fur.

When bathing your dog, use cool water. If you use the right shampoo with a good conditioner (as you do with your own hair), you can bathe him several times a week. It won't hurt him in the least—in fact his skin and coat will glow! But, be sure the shampoo you use is a moisturizing one. Dry skin is itchy and flaky, and that's a bad combination for your pet and for your allergies. Special products, such as Allergy Relief Center pet shampoo, are available that won't dry out your dog's skin and that help control dander. You can even make a homemade shampoo that works perfectly well: Combine liquid dishwashing soap, white vinegar, and glycerin. While you usually want to avoid using human shampoo on your dog, baby shampoo can work well, too.

Brushing

Brushing is another way to remove dead hair and stimulate the skin so that it remains in great condition—neither dry nor greasy. Frequent brushing helps distribute oils through the coat and reduces dander. Make every effort to find, beg, or hire someone else to brush your dog—after all, sticking your nose

BATH TIPS

- Spray your dog between baths with a moisturizer (humectant) to keep the dander down.
- If you are also allergic to grass or pollen, you might need to bathe your dog after he's been outside running around.

in dog hair isn't likely to help your allergy. If you must groom him yourself, always wear a mask and protective gloves. Use gentle strokes and avoid using any grooming tools that irritate the skin.

Dietary Care

A poor diet or one that contains ingredients to which the dog is allergic can cause the dog to have skin problems. (That's how dogs express their allergies, rather than how we do it—by sneezing.) Meat products like beef and chicken frequently cause allergies, as well as corn, wheat, and soy. Rice is much less apt to cause an allergic reaction in a dog.

Adding fatty acids to your dog's diet can help keep his skin in top shape. Omega 3 and 6 fatty acids help the skin retain moisture,

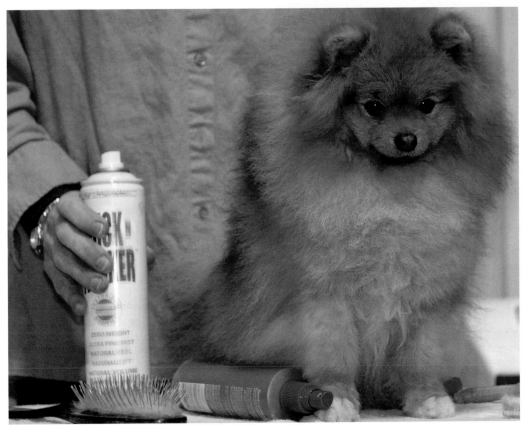

Get your spouse, friend, child, or professional groomer to groom your dog, so that you can avoid excessive contact with the dander.

Besides constant scratching, a sure of sign of fleas on your dog is the presence of blackish/reddish granules. These are flea feces, and they are largely composed of your dog's blood.

which can reduce shedding. One product I like is Mrs. Allen's Shed-Stop, a natural liquid dietary supplement with sunflower oil, vitamins, and antioxidants. Of course, it won't

A poor diet or one that contains ingredients to which the dog is allergic can cause the dog to have skin problems.

help with normal shedding, but it may work for dogs with a dietary deficiency.

Parasite Control

Skin parasites can cause itching and consequent scratching. When the dog scratches, the dander flies, the skin become more irritated, and yet more dander is produced! They key to avoiding this cycle of irritation is simple—prevent fleas, ticks, and mites from infesting your dog.

Fleas and Ticks

Nowadays, there is no excuse for your dog not to be on an anti-flea and -tick program. Flea preventives come in two basic kinds: adulticides, which, as the name suggests, kill adult fleas on contact, and insect growth regulators (IGRs), which stop little fleas from growing up into big ones and so stops the flea life cycle. (They don't kill adult fleas, though.)

Examples of adulticides are fipronil, pyrethrins, permethrin, selamectin, and imidacloprid. The first two kill ticks as well as fleas. Selamectin is kind of a "magic bullet"— it kills adult fleas and stops flea eggs from hatching. It also kills the American dog tick (but not the wood tick), ear mites, sarcoptic mange mites, and heartworm. Unlike the other chemicals, it actually enters the dog's bloodstream. IGRs include lufenuron, methoprene, and pyriproxyfen.

Ticks also can be controlled by many monthly topical insecticides (even though ticks aren't insects), such as Bio Spot for Dogs, Defend, K9 Advantix for Dogs, and Frontline Top Spot. Another kind, Revolution, contains selamectin, which, as mentioned, kills the American dog tick, among other pests. Amitraz anti-tick collars, such as Preventic, are very effective in extremely tick infested areas; they can be used in combination with a permethrin product like Biospot for optimum results. Another option is a spray that comes in an aerosol or pump bottle. Apply using a cotton ball, on the area around the ears and eyes. Most tick products contain permethrin, pyrethrin, imidacloprid, or fipronil. Read and follow the directions carefully on any preventive you use on your dog.

Use a towelette or moist wipe to remove dirt, mud, and other grime or potential allergens from your pets' paws before they can track it inside the house.

Demodectic Mange

Demodectic mange, also called red mange, is a fairly common skin disease. While the culprit, a tiny mite called *Demodex canis*, can be found on most dogs, only some seem to suffer adverse effects, which may be because of a defective immune system. Puppies are most generally affected.

The mites crowd the hair follicles, causing the hair to fall out. In addition, the follicles often become infected and the skin red and inflamed. Your vet can do a skin scraping to confirm the diagnosis. Mange in puppies usually resolves itself, but it can be also treated with insecticides.

Sarcoptic Mange

Sarcoptic mange is a highly contagious parasitic disease affecting both humans and dogs. The culprit is a microscopic mite called *Sarcoptes scabiei.* The mites burrow in the skin and cause itchiness, redness, and hair loss in both people and dogs. (This mite can affect almost any kind of animal, by the way, especially livestock.) This mange is treated with special shampoos, dips, pills, or injections. Since mange is so itchy, it plays havoc with your dog's skin, and consequently with your allergy. Take him to the vet for a check-up.

Fungal or Bacterial Infections

Fungal or bacterial infections can also make your dog scratch. Ringworm (a contagious fungus) is characterized by scabs or an irregularly shaped area of skin infection. There may be rapid hair loss at the site. It can be treated by your vet. Any bacterial infection is also likely to bother your dog.

Other Problems

Hormonal diseases like hypothyroidism can cause a drying out of the coat and consequent dander. Dogs with hypothyroidism tend to have a harsh coat with symmetrical hair loss. They are sluggish and may gain weight. Treatment is easy, effective, and inexpensive—a simple thyroid replacement pill.

Spayed and castrated dogs have fewer hormonal swings, and they tend to shed less.

Skin diseases like seborrhea can also cause skin irritation, scratching, or dander. In seborrhea, the skin produces excessive sebum, which appears as either dry flakes in the hair coat or as greasy, waxy scales on the skin. It also smells bad. Seborrhea is not really a disease in itself as much as the result of some underlying disease or condition. Once that condition is treated, the seborrhea will disappear.

The thing to remember is that any disease that makes your dog itch and scratch, or that produces excessive sebum, is going to mean more dander for him and more allergic reaction for you.

Restricting Access

It is not required for your dog to have unlimited access to every nook and cranny in your home. Keep him off furniture (especially upholstered furniture) and out of certain rooms—especially your bedroom, whether you are in it or not. Research shows that if you can breathe 8 to 10 hours of "pure" air every night, you can tolerate more exposure to allergic substances during the day. The bedroom especially should be free of clutter (including books and newspapers, rugs, drapes, junk under the bed, and so on). The more wash-

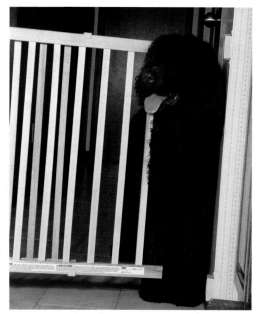

It is not required for your dog to have unlimited access to every nook and cranny in your home.

able surfaces in the room, the better.

If you do allow the dog on the couch, at least cover it with a sheet and wash the sheet every day. The sheet will collect much of the dander.

Topical Products

Some topical products work to neutralize allergens on the skin and fur. Some are sprays, others are applied with a cloth to the fur. Some products require daily application; others can be used less often. They also take some time to take effect.

After brushing or a bath, you can finish off using an anti-allergy product like Allerpet/D, by Nature's Miracle. (There's an Allerpet/C for cats.) Just apply with a damp cloth, and pay special attention to those spots the dog licks most often. During dry spells,

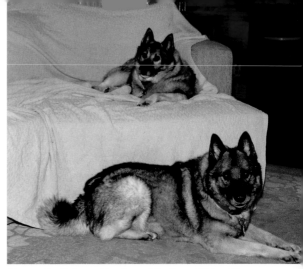

If you don't have the heart to keep Fido off the couch, at least cover it with a sheet and wash the sheet every day.

spray a bit of Allerpet or a similar substance on the dog's coat to keep the dander produced from flying all over the house.

Nature's Miracle also produces Nature's Miracle Dander Remover and Deodorizer,

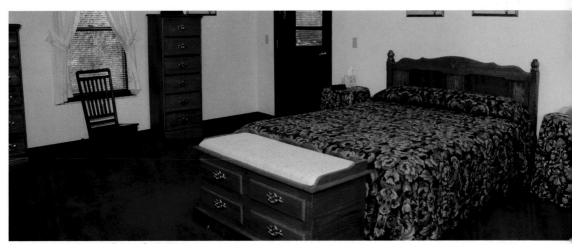

Keep the bedroom free of clutter.

In rare cases, repeated flare-up of allergy attacks in children can cause lung damage. In cases like this, you may be forced to find the pet another home if you can't bring the allergy under control.

Allerpet Allergy Relief, and Outright Allergy Relief. These nontoxic, nonstaining liquids are applied topically to the pet: Rub in and wipe off to clean away dander and soften the pet's skin so that less dander is produced.

Another excellent product is the British-made Petal Cleanse/D for dogs. It is a clear, colorless liquid that removes the dander and other allergens from the coat and encapsulates them. It contains moisturizers that condition the coat and skin to further reduce the amount of material shed.

Toy and Dog Bedding Care

Wash all dog toys and bedding frequently in soapy water of at least 103°F (39.4°C). Your dog's bedding should be covered in allergen-resistant plastic. There's even an allergen-resistant dog bed, made from "breathable" Cordura nylon, a washable fabric tougher than cotton or fleece, that traps dust and other allergy-causing particles.

Wash Your Clothing (And Yourself!)

After grooming or playing with your dog, remove your clothing, which will be full of animal dander, and wash it. Keep these clothes out of the bedroom—bring them straight to the washing machine. Wash your face, hands, and arms, too. Do not touch your face, especially your eyes, until after you have done so.

TO PREVENT YOUR CHILD FROM DEVELOPING AN ALLERGY—GET A PET

A 2001 Swedish study has shown that very early exposure (during infancy) to animals may reduce the chances that a child will develop allergies later in life. Four hundred and twelve children were tested for allergies at age 7 years and again at age 12. Of those children who were not around cats or dogs during their first year, nearly 9 percent developed asthma, compared to only 3 percent of children who were exposed to pets. Allergies also developed in nearly 9 percent of children in the no-pet group, while only 6 percent of the pet-exposed children did.

Another, larger Swedish study, done in 2003, by allergist Thomas Platts-Mills of the University of Virginia and Swedish researchers, found that, out of the 2,500 children they studied, the longer children had pets—ideally during their first 2 years—the lower their fre-

I know it's hard, but please do not hug or kiss your dog if you suffer dog-dander allergies.

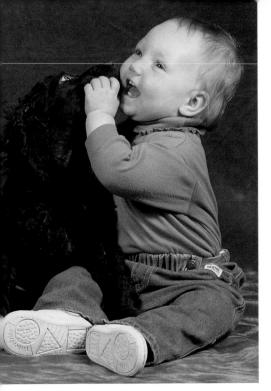

A study has shown that very early exposure to animals may reduce the chances that a child will develop allergies later in life.

quency of having pet allergies. Children who continually owned pets were less likely to have pet dander allergies than new pet owners or those who had been exposed only earlier in life. In fact, of those who proved to be allergic to cats, 80% never had a cat at home.

In 2002, another study found that babies raised in a home with two or more dogs or cats were up to 77% less likely to develop various types of allergies at age 6 than kids raised without pets. The protective effect worked not only against pet dander allergies,

but against other kinds as well, such as allergies to dust mites, ragweed, and grass.

One explanation is that early high pet-allergen exposure may lead to changes in the immune system so that it is less likely to produce an allergic response.

Dennis R. Ownby, chief of Allergy and Immunology at the Medical College of Georgia, studied 474 children from birth to age 7. He discovered that children exposed to two or more indoor pets were less than half as likely to develop allergies—not just to pet secretions, but also to ragweed, dust mites, and grass. Ownby theorizes that the licks children receive when playing with their pets transfer enough gram-negative bacteria to change the way the child's immune system responds. However, be forewarned: Parents who smoke wipe out the anti-allergy benefits their infants receive from early pet exposure.

DON'T FORGET

- Dog allergies can be controlled!
- Treat *yourself* with immunotherapy, antihistamines, eyedrops, and nasal sprays.
- Treat the *house* by cleaning, vacuuming, using hypoallergenic materials, and keeping the bedroom dog-free.
- Treat the *dog* by bathing, wipes, getting someone else to help, and keeping your dog healthy.

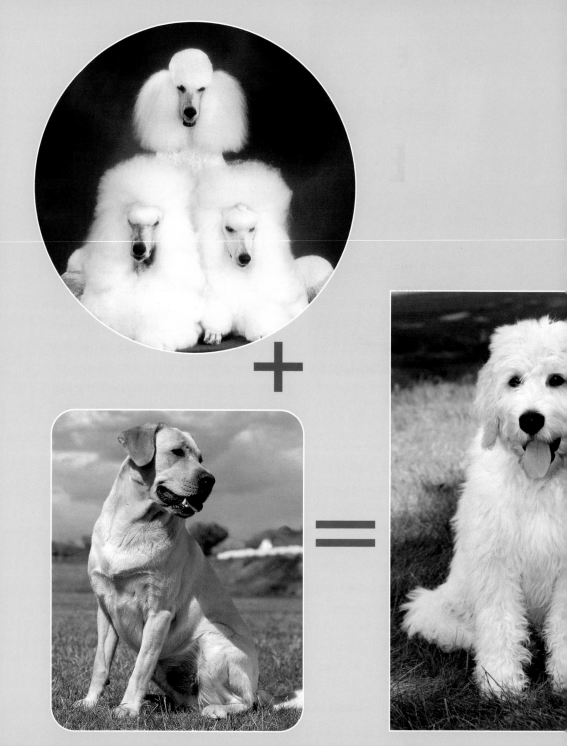

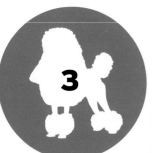

Beyond the Hype in

Hypoallergenic Breeds

3

ALL OVER THE INTERNET, AND IN COUNTLESS NEWS STORIES and rumors, we hear about hypoallergenic dogs—dogs who don't cause an allergic reaction. Alas, if only it were completely true. The fact is that no such breed exists, if by "hypoallergenic" we mean a dog who cannot provoke an allergy in any single person. Such an animal would have no hair, no dander, no saliva, and no urine. And believe me, when someone develops a urine-free dog, more people than allergy sufferers will be anxious to get one!

Different people are allergic to different proteins and so, while some people might have no symptoms from a hairless dog, others who are allergic to proteins in the saliva will be just as allergic as ever. All dogs (including hairless ones) produce dander, and all dogs have saliva. All dogs urinate. However, it is true that some breeds, because they are low-shedding or have a single coat, are less apt to cause severe symptoms than are hairier, heavier-coated breeds.

DESIGNER DOGS

Do not believe claims that someone has developed a designer or nonallergenic dog. While there have been several attempts to develop a truly allergy-free breed, this effort has not met with notable success. They do not exist, and cannot exist, until someone makes a dog without saliva, urine, or dander. The so-called designer dogs are nothing more than ordinary mixes, in which (the breeder hopes) the desirable characteristics of two breeds are combined. Thus, the Labradoodle is supposed to have Poodle-like hair and a Labrador temperament. The Labraddoodle may well have inherited some of the hypoallergenic qualities of the Poodle, but they are not any more hypoallergenic than a purebred Poodle. So far, none of the "manufactured breeds" are any less allergenic than those mentioned in the next chapter.

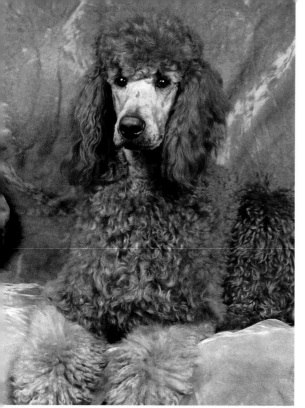

Cross-breeders use Poodles for their hypoallergenic qualities.

In addition, as of this writing, these "breeds" are still not "breeding true." In dog breeding, "breeding true" means that the progeny closely resemble their parents—this is how new breeds are developed and eventually officially acknowledged. Therefore, these crosses cannot yet count as "real" breeds. Stay tuned.

Dog Crossbreeds

Labradoodles were initially bred by the Australian Guide Dogs Association in an attempt to produce a "hypoallergenic" guide dog. They have had a lot of publicity in Australia, and are widely believed to be hypoallergenic. However, this is not universally the case. The hair on a Labradoodle is not the same as Poodle wool.

According to the Guide dog breeders, some first-cross Labradoodles appear to be hypoallergenic. Labradoodle guide dogs have been tested against their potential owners, and some dogs have been placed with people with allergies, at least right now.

Several other interesting mixes are sometimes touted as "new breeds," but most of them are just crossbreeds. There's nothing wrong with this, but you shouldn't be duped into paying an exorbitant price for a nonpedigreed dog (unless he's a movie actor or formerly owned by Britney Spears). To date, no crossbred dog is more allergenic than its more allergenic parent—or more hypoallergenic than its more hypoallergenic parent. So, a Labradoodle won't be any more hypoallergenic than a Poodle. Now if you have a "Maltipoo" (half poodle and half Maltese), you have a fairly good hypoallergenic cross. But beware of anything with "Cocker Spaniel" in the cross. There's a ton of loose hair on those dogs.....

THE INDIVIDUAL DIFFERENCES

Some recent studies suggest that differences between individual dogs (even dogs from the same litter) may be greater than that

Some breeds have breed-specific allergens—so someone allergic to a Basenji may be just fine around a Chinese Crested.

between different breeds. An allergic person may react to one dog (even a hairless one) but perhaps not to another individual, even if the latter is from a breed not normally termed hypoallergenic.

Individual pets produce individual amounts of dander. In addition, it has been discovered that several breeds do have breed-specific allergens! So, you might be allergic to Basenjis, but not to Chinese Cresteds, or vice versa.

"HYPOALLERGENIC" BREEDS

So, now we know that there is no such thing as a totally *nonallergenic* breed of dog. So, what's an allergy sufferer to do? Some breeds, often touted as "hypoallergenic," may not affect allergy-prone people as much because of the type of hair they have or amount they shed. These breeds include:

- **Curly-coated breeds** like Poodles, Bichon Frises, Portuguese Water Dogs, Pulik, Komondorak, and Irish Water Spaniels.
- **Hairless breeds** like Xoloitzcuintli, Chinese Cresteds, American Hairless Terriers, and Peruvian Inca Orchids.

- **Low-shedding or single-coated breeds** like Basenjis, Coton du Tulear, Chihuahuas, Italian Greyhounds, and Maltese.

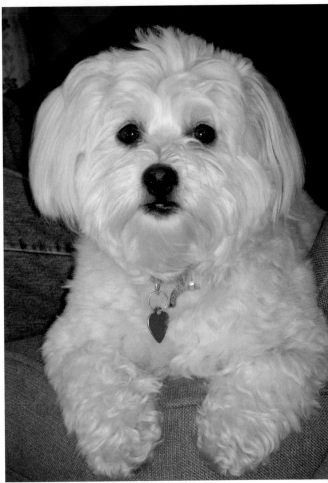

A Maltipoo is a good hypoallergenic cross.

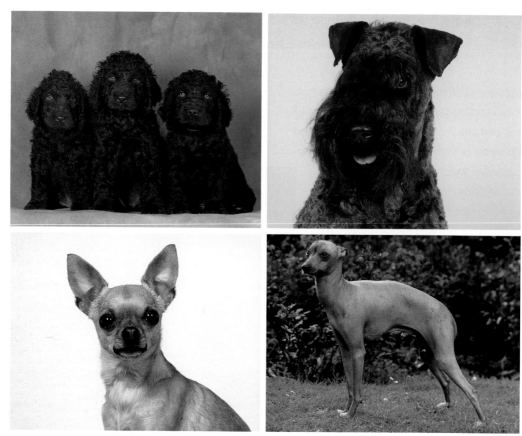

Curly-coated, terrier-type, low-shedding, and hairless breeds tend to be better for allergy sufferers.

- **Terrier-type breeds** like Schnauzers, Bedlington Terriers, Soft-Coated Wheaten Terriers, and Kerry Blue Terriers.

Why might these dogs be better than others? Some of the secret is in the hair, and the rule is simple: Dogs whose hair falls out a lot tend to trigger allergies in their owners. The reverse is also true—dogs who do not shed much or have much hair to shed won't trigger as many allergies. Curly-coated and wirehaired breeds tend to shed very little—they have a long growth cycle to their hair. Hairless dogs have no hair (although they still produce dander). So, these types of dogs may be for someone who is prone to allergies.

Care Considerations

Many "hypoallergenic" breeds do require considerable care. Terriers and curly-coated breeds need lots of clipping and coat care.

It is possible that female dogs produce fewer allergens than do males. We know this is true of cats, but sufficient studies have not yet been done with dogs.

The Komondor and Puli have corded coats like dreadlocks that are extremely difficult to maintain. Hairless breeds need diligent skin care, and protection from the sun and cold elements. Some single-coated breeds like Maltese, have easily matted and tangled hair.

Think Small

All things being equal, think small. Smaller dogs produce much less hair and less dander than big ones. Younger animals also produce less dander and have softer and more pliant skin than older ones. So, you may

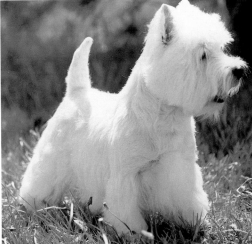

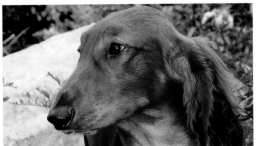

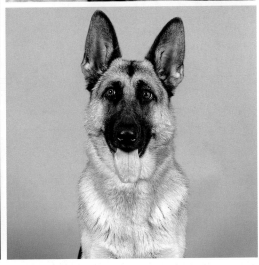

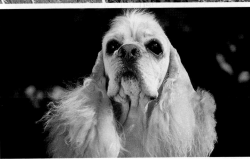

Breeds like the West Highland White Terrier, Dachshund, Cocker Spaniel and German Shepherd tend to produce a lot of dander.

not be allergic to your puppy, but become allergic to him as he ages. (Best to start with an older dog in the first place to avoid any potential heartbreak.)

Dog Don'ts

The following breeds produce lots of dander and tend to be especially troublesome for allergy sufferers:

- Afghan Hounds
- Basset Hounds
- Chinese Shar-Peis
- Cocker Spaniels (both types)
- Dachshunds
- Doberman Pinschers
- German Shepherd Dogs
- Irish Setters
- Springer Spaniel (both types)
- West Highland White Terriers

In fact, these same breeds often have skin problems themselves. These breeds frequently suffer from dry or oily seborrhea that makes the skin cells turn over at a rapid rate—every few days instead of every few weeks. This doesn't mean you

> If you are allergic to the saliva of dogs, it doesn't matter how much hair the dog has or doesn't have, or what kind of hair it is.

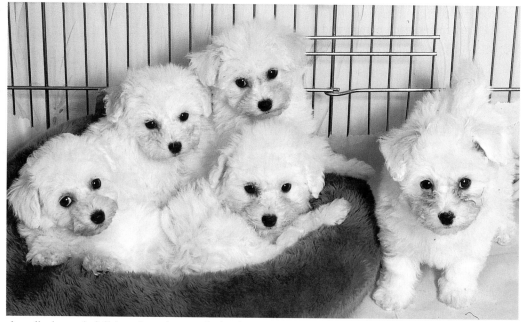

A well-planned visit to a breeder can help give you a hint about how you will react to a dog.

Another great option is to volunteer as a foster home for an all-breed dog rescue organization. You'll get all kinds of experience with all kinds of breeds. One of them is sure to be right for you!

can't own one of these breeds, but it does mean you have to be super-vigilant about maintaining him (or having him maintained).

Finding Fido

So, now you know a bit about how allergies work and what you can do can do to manage them. The next chapter lists those breeds that, as a group, tend to provoke fewer reactions among allergy-sensitive people that others.

Just remember, each person and each dog is an individual. You may be allergic to the most hypoallergenic of dogs, or you may not be. And, unfortunately, too, you may be nonallergic to most individuals of a particular breed and react badly to just the one you decide to bring home. But, life is a risk and, as we discussed in the previous chapter, most people can manage to keep their dog—even if they don't completely conquer their allergy.

While nothing substitutes for actually having a dog in your home for an extended period, you can get

some hint about how you will react from a well-planned visit. Make an appointment and go directly to the breeder's house without visiting any other dogs on the way.

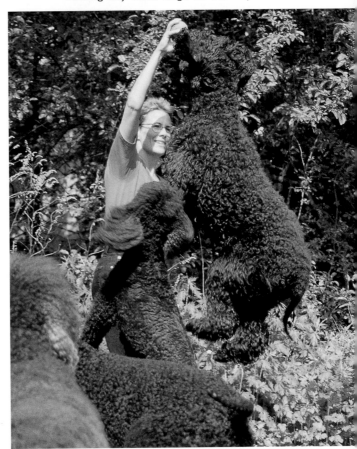

Besides a dog's hypo-allergenic properties, you'll have to consider things like activity level.

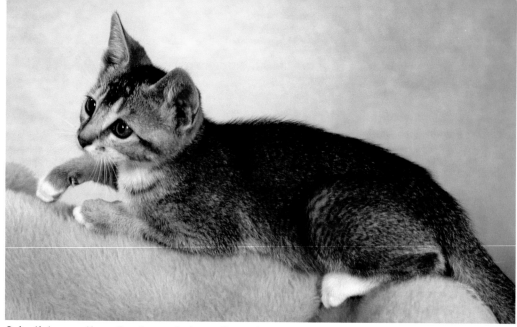
Scientists are attempting to create hypoallergenic cats.

The breeder should only have one breed of dog living in that house; otherwise, if you are allergic, the test is inconclusive (it might have been a reaction to the other breed). The visit should take place in an area where no other animals or allergens are present. Spend at least 1 or 2 hours with the dog—then leave. Do not visit any other dogs for several hours, to eliminate the possibility of a delayed reaction. Repeat the visit as often as you can. The allergic person should hold the dog for several minutes during the visit.

With careful breed selection and home management, you can be on your way to one of the 69.1 million homes who enjoy a loving family dog.

GENETICALLY ENGINEERED HYPOALLERGENIC CATS: CAN DOGS BE FAR BEHIND?

Perhaps the ultimate answer lies in technology. While no "natural" cat breed is truly hypoallergenic, a California biotechnology company, Allerca, has started taking orders for a hypoallergenic cat for pet lovers prone to allergies.

The first genetically engineered feline is expected to be available in early 2007. Using "gene silencing" technology, Allerca is able to suppress the production of the protein responsible for cat allergy. Allerca president Simon Brodie says he ultimately hopes to sell 200,000 of the cats annually, at $3,500 each, in the United States. (The cats

With careful breed selection and home management, you can be on your way to welcoming a dog in the family

will be neutered before sale, for obvious reasons.)

The first breed of hypoallergenic cats will be British Shorthairs, who are friendly, affectionate, and playful cats. Even this cat, however, is not allergy free. It simply produces much less allergen. Brodie explains: "It's like hypoallergenic makeup. The allergens are still there, but in very small amounts that don't trigger allergic reactions." And what do the experts say?

"I have my doubts that this is going to work," David Rosenstreich, M.D., director of allergy and immunology at Albert Einstein School of Medicine in New York. "Fel-d1 is the major protein that patients are also allergic to. But there are other proteins that cats produce that people are allergic to. Getting rid of Fel-d1 will not create a completely nonallergenic cat."

Dr. Gailen Marshall, director of clinical immunology and allergy at the University of Mississippi Medical Center, adds, "I'm not sure I like the idea of genetically manipulated cats, but I'll keep an open mind to it....It could be problematic over time. The allergen protein is very stable; it lives for long periods of time. This cat will still have dander, still groom itself, still have a kitty litter box. That cumulative amount could become an allergy issue—it's simply delayed rather than eliminated."

DON'T FORGET

- The so-called "designer dog" is a fancy name for a cross-breed.
- The most popular "designer dog" is the Labradoodle, a cross between a Poodle and a Labrador Retriever.
- A Labradoodle is about as hypoallergenic as its Poodle parent, but gets more fanfare.
- Among recognized breeds, curly-coated, hairless, and wire-coated breeds tend to trigger fewer allergies than other dogs.
- It's all individual. Not all allergic people respond the same way to the different breeds, or even to different dogs within the same breed.
- Don't give up. Your own hypoallergenic dog may be out there looking for you.

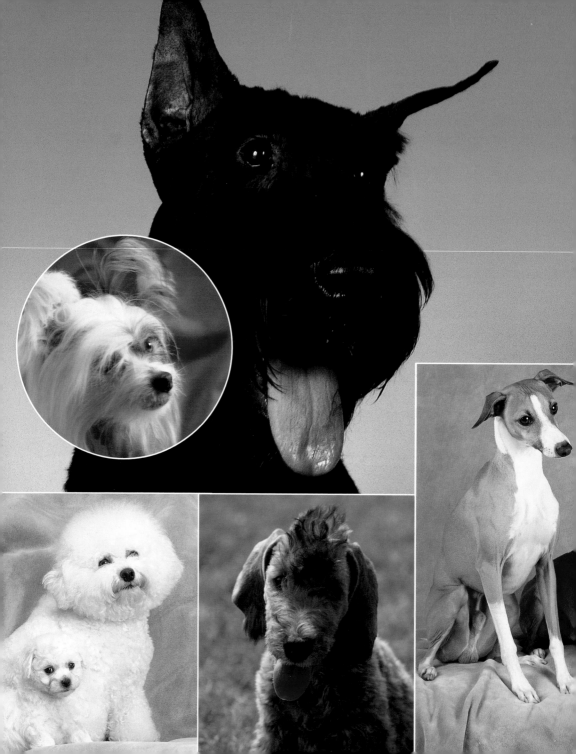

Meet the Breeds

4

I N THIS SECTION, WE'RE GOING TO TAKE A LOOK at some of the most "hypoallergenic breeds." But, whether or not a dog is hypoallergenic cannot be your only consideration in choosing a breed. The breed's size, activity level, trainability, habits, and other factors should be equally important factors in your decision.

First a note: Every dog is an individual. I may list a breed as "low" in trainability, but this does not mean that your dog will be hard to train. Nor does it mean that the breed in general is not trainable; it simply means that it may take more patience than with other breeds. It certainly does not mean the dog is dumb—wolves are incredibly intelligent and notoriously untrainable. Trainability has more to do with compliance than brilliance.

The same goes for the other traits I list. Some members of "highly active" breeds are couch potatoes, and vice versa. Please consider the Vital Statistics section as general guidelines, not facts carved in stone.

You will notice lots of health problems listed for most breeds. That does not mean that your dog is likely to get all (or even any) of them. It merely means that these problems have been noted in the breed.

That being said, it is important to understand that different breeds were bred for different purposes, and most breed characteristics relate to those original purposes. Many characteristics cannot be "trained out" of breeds, although some can be managed. Thus, it is very important to look beyond "hypoallergenic qualities" and even size when hunting for that "perfect dog." Read the breed profiles carefully and see if the named dog matches your needs. It's best to find out these things before you get the dog—not after.

PART 1
CURLY-COATED AND CORDED BREEDS

Curly-coated and Corded breeds do shed, but their hair has a long life-span, so shedding is infrequent. In addition, the shed hair doesn't fly around the room, but clings to the cords that naturally form on the dog, thus producing fewer allergy symptoms than most other breeds.

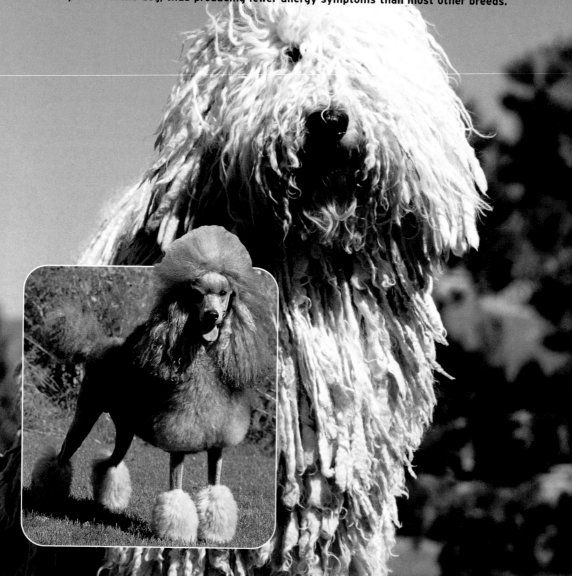

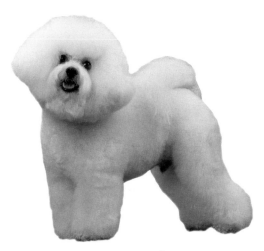

BICHON FRISE

This Mediterranean breed is descended from the Barbet, or Water Spaniel, and the Bichon is related to the Poodle and Maltese, two other "hypoallergenic" breeds. While a long-time favorite in Italy, the Bichon reached the peak of his popularity in France, where it said that Henri III (1574–1589) was so enchanted by his Bichon that he carried him wherever he went in a tray-like basket attached around his neck by ribbons. The Spanish painter Goya must have been inordinately fond of this breed, considering how often he painted them. Perhaps Goya had an allergy to other dogs, one never knows (or nose). Titian and Joshua Reynolds also painted the breed.

The words *Bichon Frise* mean "curly-coated lap dog." The French nobility took a liking to them, but during the Revolution, many were tossed out on the street, where only the toughest survived. Many of them worked the streets as assistants to organ grinders. Some got jobs in the circus, and still others led

BICHON TIP

The Bichon Frise Club of America advises: "Experience shows that those with mild allergies may be able to share a home with a Bichon. The person with severe allergies may be at risk for a severe attack when exposed to these dogs. Others will fall between those parameters. If you do decide to buy the Bichon, realize that adult coats are different from puppy coats, so allergic individual should be exposed to both."

Activity Level:

Low = **Couch potato alert! But remember even low-energy dogs still need moderate exercise.**

Medium = **Fairly active. Should be moderately to heavily exercised once or twice a day.**

High = **You've got an Energizer Bunny on your hands. Serious exercise is needed daily or you could end up with behavior problems.**

Trainability:

Low = **May need some extra time and attention with training.**

Medium = **Should pick up basic training fairly easily.**

High = **He's a pleaser! Will most likely pick up training easily.**

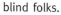

blind folks.

The Bichon Frise is a cheerful, friendly little dog. In fact, of all small dogs, I would rate the Bichon one of the most outgoing and friendly with new people. He demands a lot of attention from his owner, but will reward you with his playful antics.

Vital Statistics

National Club: Bichon Frise Club of America. Visit them at www.bichon.org.

Origin: Mediterranean region, probably the Canary Islands in the 1300s.

Group: Non-Sporting (AKC)/Toy (KC)

Size: 9 to 12 inches (30 cm); 7 to 12 pounds (3 to 5 kg).

Lifespan: 13 to 15 years.

Colors: White. Puppies may have traces of buff, cream, or apricot.

Grooming: The fluffy coat requires frequent brushing, preferably every day. Their coat is somewhat silkier than the Poodle's, with the outer coat coarser and curlier than the inner one. Although the breed seldom sheds, dead hair of the undercoat must be combed out frequently to prevent mats and hot spots.

Personality: Friendly, cheerful, playful, bold, happy-go-lucky.

Sociability: Excellent with older children and pets. They bond with the whole family, but some are too sensitive for toddlers.

Activity Level: Low to Medium.

Trainability: High. Housetraining problems have been observed in a few.

Health Issues: Skin and allergy problems (this hypoallergenic dogs is prone to allergies itself); ear infections, dental problems (early tooth loss, tartar) eye problems (cataracts), bladder stones and infections, luxating patella, involuntary movement disorder, and diseases of the endocrine system (pancreatitis, Cushing's, and diabetes). Note: Talk to your vet about a vaccination protocol for this breed, which may be different from that of others.

Adoption Option: If you are interested in adopting a Bichon Frise in need, contact www.bichon.org/usrescueeffort.htm. The U.S. Bichon Frise Rescue Effort is a nationwide volunteer program with currently over 30 active "Rescue Representatives." The program works in conjunction with the national breed parent club, the Bichon Frise Club of America.

Breed Standard in Brief

(Adapted from the Bichon Frise Club of America)

General Appearance: The Bichon Frise is a small, sturdy, white powder puff of a dog. His merry temperament is expressed by his plumed tail carried jauntily over the back and his dark-eyed, inquisitive expression. He should be compact and of medium bone, neither coarse nor fine.

Size, Proportion, Substance: The preference is for animals 9.5 to 11.5 inches (24 to 29 cm). In proportion, body from the forward-most point of the chest to the point of rump is one-quarter longer than the height at the

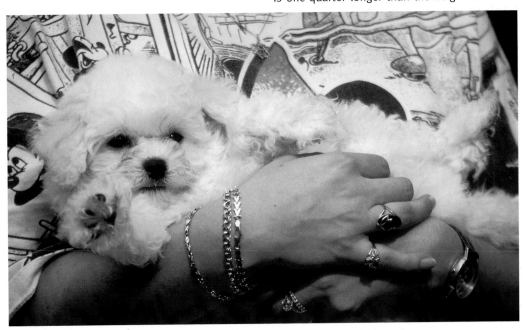

The words Bichon Frise mean "curly-coated lap dog."

withers. The body from the withers to lowest point of chest represents half the distance from withers to ground.

Head: The expression is soft, dark-eyed, inquisitive, and alert. The eyes are round, black or dark brown, and are set in the skull to look directly forward. An overly large or bulging eye or an almond-shaped, obliquely set eye is a fault. Halos, the black or very dark brown skin surrounding the eyes, are necessary, as they accentuate the eye and enhance expression. The eye rims themselves must be black. Broken pigment, or total absence of pigment on the eye rims, is a definite fault. Eyes of any color other than black or dark brown are a very serious fault and must be severely penalized in the show ring. The ears are drop and are covered with long flowing hair. When extended toward the nose, the leathers reach approximately halfway the length of the muzzle. They are set on slightly higher than eye level and rather forward on the skull. The skull is slightly rounded. The stop is slightly accentuated. A properly balanced head is three parts muzzle to five parts skull, measured from the nose to the stop and from the stop to the occiput. There is a slight degree of chiseling under the eyes, but not so much as to result in a weak or snipey foreface. The lower jaw is strong. The nose is prominent and always black. The lips are black, fine, never drooping. The bite is scissors. A bite which is undershot or overshot should be severely penalized. A crooked or out of line tooth is permissible; however, missing teeth are to be severely faulted.

Neck, Topline, and Body: The arched neck is long and carried proudly behind an erect head. It blends smoothly into the shoulders. The length of neck from occiput to withers is approximately one-third the distance from forechest to buttocks. The topline is level except for a slight, muscular arch over the loin. The chest is well developed and wide enough to allow free and unrestricted movement of the front legs. The lowest point of the chest extends at least to the elbow. The rib cage is moderately sprung and extends back to a short and muscular loin. The forechest is pronounced and protrudes slightly forward of the point of shoulder. The underline has a moderate tuck-up. The tail is well plumed, set on level with the topline and curved gracefully over the back so that the hair of the tail rests on the back. When the tail is extended toward the head it reaches at least halfway to the withers. A low tail set, a tail carried perpendicularly to the back, or a tail which droops behind is to be severely penalized. A corkscrew tail is a very serious fault.

Forequarters: The shoulder blade, upper arm, and forearm are approximately equal in length. The shoulders are laid back to near a forty-five degree angle. The upper arm extends

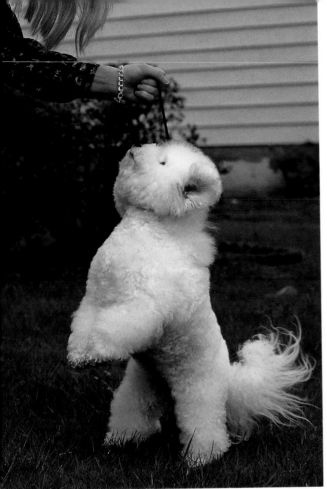

Bichons are usually highly trainable.

point directly forward, turning neither in nor out. Pads are black. Nails are kept short.

Hindquarters: The hindquarters are of medium bone, well angulated with muscular thighs and spaced moderately wide. The upper and lower thigh are nearly equal in length, meeting at a well bent stifle joint. The leg from hock joint to foot pad is perpendicular to the ground. Dewclaws may be removed. Paws are tight and round with black pads.

Coat: The texture of the coat is of utmost importance. The undercoat is soft and dense, the outer coat of a coarser and curlier texture. The combination of the two gives a soft but substantial feel to the touch, which is similar to plush or velvet and, when patted, springs back. When bathed and brushed, it stands off the body, creating an overall powder puff appearance. A wiry coat is not desirable. A limp, silky coat, a coat that lies down, or a lack of undercoat are very serious faults. The coat is trimmed to reveal the natural outline of the body. It is rounded off from any direction and never cut so short as to create an overly trimmed or squared off appearance. The furnishings of the head, beard, moustache, ears, and tail are left

well back, so the elbow is placed directly below the withers when viewed from the side. The legs are of medium bone; straight, with no bow or curve in the forearm or wrist. The elbows are held close to the body. The pasterns slope slightly from the vertical. The dewclaws may be removed. The feet are tight and round, resembling those of a cat and

longer. The longer head hair is trimmed to create an overall rounded impression. The topline is trimmed to appear level. The coat is long enough to maintain the powder puff look which is characteristic of the breed.

Color: Color is white, may have shadings of buff, cream, or apricot around the ears or on the body. Any color in excess of 10% of the entire coat of a mature specimen is a fault and should be penalized, but color of the accepted shadings should not be faulted in puppies.

Gait: Movement at a trot is free, precise, and effortless. In profile, the forelegs and hind legs extend equally with an easy reach and drive that maintain a steady topline. When moving, the head and neck remain somewhat erect and, as speed increases, there is a very slight convergence of legs toward the center line. Moving away, the hindquarters travel with moderate width between them and the foot pads can be seen.

Temperament: Gentle mannered, sensitive, playful, and affectionate. A cheerful attitude is the hallmark of the breed and one should settle for nothing less.

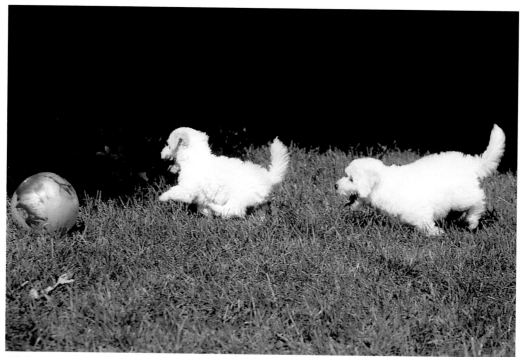

Bichons are known for their cheerful attitudes.

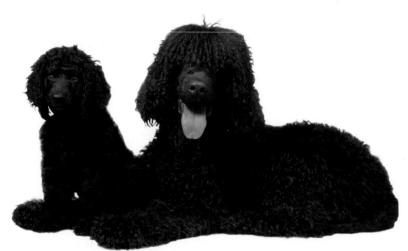

IRISH WATER SPANIEL

Once known as Shannon, Rat-tail, or Whip-Tail Spaniels, the Irish Water Spaniel (IWS) is sometimes confused with the Poodle, although there are important differences between the two breeds. (Some experts believe the Poodle was one ancestor of the breed; others have tapped the Afghan.) The IWS has a whiplike, bare, rather than docked tail, and the face is entirely and naturally smooth-coated. Like many water dogs, he has webbed toes. This breed is not a barker. This super hunting dog works on upland game as well as waterfowl, making him an excellent dual-purpose dog.

The IWS is considered "hypoallergenic" partly because of his hair texture, which, according to the IWS website, prevents the coat from becoming tightly woven into fabric and upholstery; any stray hairs are easily removed, because they will gather together to form "dust bunnies."

> The Irish Water Spaniel is the tallest of the spaniels (and is sometimes confused with a Poodle, although the tails are very different).

Vital Statistics

National Breed Club: Irish Water Spaniel Club of America. Visit them at www.clubs.akc.org/iwsc.

Origin: Ireland. The recognizable forebears of the breed date back to the 1100s.

Group: Sporting Group (AKC)/Gundog (KC)

Size: 21 to 24 inches (53 to 61 cm); 45 to 65 pounds (20 to 29 kg).

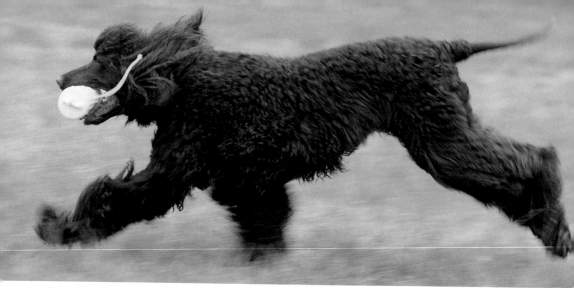

Irish Water Spaniels need lots of exercise.

Lifespan: 10 to 12 years.

Colors: Liver.

Grooming: Tight curls, negligible shedding. The coat must be kept mat-free by regular combing, and requires scissoring, which will be required every 6 to 8 weeks to neaten and shape the coat. Regular exposure to water will promote the correct "ringlets" over the body coat. Needs professional grooming, and gives off a characteristic smell due to the somewhat oily coat.

Personality: Playful, willing, active, gentle, exuberant.

Sociability: Somewhat standoffish. May not get along with other pets. Requires early socialization.

Activity Level: High.

Trainability: High.

Health Issues: Hip dysplasia, hypothyroidism, entropion, seizures. Skin and coat problems. Von Willebrand's disease, autoimmune diseases. Some are sensitive to ivermectin, sulfa drugs, and certain anesthesia.

Adoption Option: For information about Irish Water Spaniel breed rescue and its policies, please visit them at: www.clubs.akc.org/iwsc/Rescue/contacts.htm.

Breed Standard in Brief

(Adapted from the Irish Water Spaniel Club of America)

General Appearance: The Irish Water Spaniel presents a picture of a smart, upstanding, strongly built sporting dog. Distinguishing characteristics are a topknot of long, loose curls, a body covered with a dense, crisply curled liver-colored coat, contrasted by a smooth face and a smooth "rat" tail.

Size, Proportion, Substance: Strongly built and well boned, the Irish Water Spaniel is a dog of medium length, slightly rectangular in appearance. He is well balanced, and shows no legginess or coarseness. Males 22 to 24 inches (56 to 61 cm), females 21 to 23 inches (53 to 58 cm), measured at the highest point of the shoulder. Males 55 to 65 pounds (25 to 29 kg), females 45 to 58 pounds (20 to 26 kg).

Head: The head is cleanly chiseled. The skull is rather large and high in the dome, with a prominent occiput and a gradual stop. The muzzle is square and rather long. The nose is large and liver in color. Teeth are strong and regular with a scissors or level bite. The hair on the face is short and smooth, except for a beard, which grows in a narrow line at the back of the jaw. The topknot is a characteristic of the breed, and consists of long, loose curls growing down into a well-defined peak between the eyes and falling like a shawl over the tops of the ears and occiput. Trimming of this breed characteristic in an exaggerated manner is highly objectionable. The eyes are medium in size, slightly almond-shaped, with tight eyelids. Eyes are hazel in color, preferably of a dark shade. The expression is keenly alert, intelligent, direct, and quizzical. The ears are long, lobular, set low, with leathers reaching about to the end of the nose when extended forward, and abundantly covered with long curls, extending two or more inches below the tips of the leathers.

Neck, Topline, Body: The neck is long, arching, strong, and muscular; smoothly set into shoulders. The topline is level, or slightly higher in the rear. The body is of medium length, slightly rectangular. Chest deep, with brisket extending to the elbows. Ribs well sprung and carried well back. Immediately behind the shoulders, ribs are flattened enough to allow free movement of the forelegs, becoming rounder behind. Loin short, wide, and muscular.

Forequarters: The entire front gives the impression of strength without heaviness. Shoulders are sloping and clean. Forelegs well boned, muscular, medium in length; with sufficient length of upper arm to ensure efficient reach. Elbows close set. Forefeet are large, thick, and somewhat spreading; well clothed with hair both over and between the toes.

Hindquarters: Hindquarters are as high as or slightly higher than the shoulders, powerful and muscular. Hips wide, stifles moderately bent, hocks low set and moderately bent. Rear angulation is moderate, and balance of front and rear angulation is of paramount importance. Rear feet are large, thick, and somewhat spreading; well clothed with hair. Tail should be set on low enough to give a rather rounded appearance to the hindquarters and should be carried nearly level with the back.

Tail: The so-called "rat tail" is a striking characteristic of the breed. At the root, it is thick and covered for 2 or 3 inches (5 to 8 cm) with short curls. It tapers to a fine point at the end; and from the root curls is covered with short, smooth hair so as to look as if it had been clipped. The tail should not be long enough to reach the hock joint.

Coat: The Irish Water Spaniel has a double coat. The neck, back, sides, and rear are densely covered with tight, crisp ringlets, with the hair longer underneath the ribs. Forelegs are well covered with abundant curls or waves. The hind legs should also be abundantly covered by hair falling in curls or waves, except that the hair should be short and smooth on the front of the legs below the hocks. The hair on the throat is very short and smooth, forming a V-shaped patch. All curled areas should be clearly defined by curls of sufficient length to form a sharp contrast with the smooth coat on face, throat, tail, and rear legs below the hocks. Fore and hind feet should be well clothed with hair both over and between the toes.

Color: Solid liver.

Gait: The Irish Water Spaniel moves with a smooth, free, ground-covering action that, when viewed from the side, exhibits balanced reach and drive. When walking or standing, the legs are perpendicular to the ground, toeing neither in nor out.

Temperament: Very alert and inquisitive, the Irish Water Spaniel is often reserved with strangers. However, aggressive behavior or excessive shyness should be penalized.

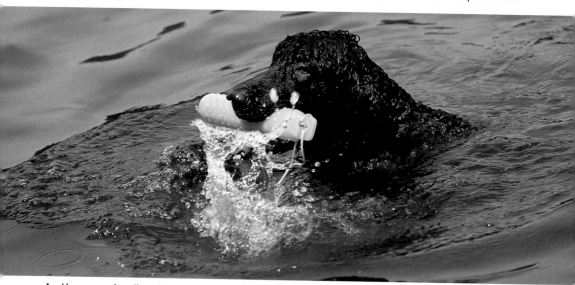

As the name implies, the Irish Water Spaniel makes a superb water dog.

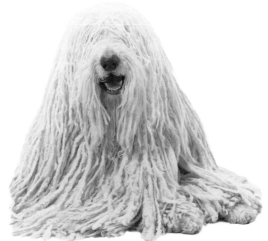

KOMONDOR

The Komondor is known as the King of the Hungarian livestock guarding dogs. The Magyars brought this dog to Hungary from the steppes of Russia, although their ancestors probably hail from Tibet (it's hard to know just where the Magyars picked them up). The Komondor is a flock guardian (not a herding dog like a collie), guarding his charges from wolves, feral dogs, and even human predators.

The plural of Komondor is Komondorak.

This is a job that requires a calm, watchful demeanor and independent thinking and action. Commands from the owner were not necessary (and, in fact, the owner was seldom around). To this day, the Komondor possesses this guarding tendency, and will select his family for his "herd." This dog is not naturally obedient, and he is very independent. He requires firm (not harsh), consistent handling by an experienced dog-person. This is not a dog for a beginner, or indeed for anyone who is not committed to caring for his complicated coat and dealing with his unusual and powerful personality.

This big, muscular dog does not tolerate heat well (it doesn't get hot in Tibet or Russia), although the cold does not affect him. Some Komondorak are quite barky.

One of the Komondor's most striking features is his corded coat. The cords both insulate and cool, and open to the skin so that they allow air to pass through. The cords form when the woolly undercoat is "trapped" by the harsh, curly outer coat. As the coat begins to mat together, the curl of the outer coat helps determine the natural separation points.

Vital Statistics

National Club: Komondor Club of America. Visit them at www.clubs.akc.org/kca/index.htm.

Origin: Hungary, antiquity. Ancestors probably hailed from Tibet.

Group: Herding (AKC)/Pastoral (KC).

Size: 25 to31 inches (63 to 79 cm); 60 to 130 pounds (27 to 59 kg).

Lifespan: 12 years.

Colors: White.

Grooming: Ground-length corded, weather-resistant coat. Nonshedding, but the coat tends to knot. Hair grows in between the pads of the toes, and requires regular trimming. They require careful ear care, too. This dog is a major challenge to bathe and dry! When not properly cared for, the coat can mat and start to smell bad.

Personality: Serious, aloof, bold, territorial, challenging.

Sociability: Tends to be a one-person or family dog. Not especially good with strange children, aloof to strangers, many be aggressive to other breeds. He will protect his family, including cats, against all perceived enemies. They have been known to crash through windows protecting their own. Early socialization is very important.

Activity Level: High, but usually quiet around the house.

KOMONDOR GROOMING TIP

The Komondor Club of America has this tip for Komondor groomers. "Separate the clumps following the pattern of the curls, having the base of the cords approximately the size of a quarter. With time and the process of wetting and drying, the clumps will tighten up, forming cords. At first, these cords will be short, but as the dog ages, the coat grows longer, the cords will acquire the length and graceful swing of the impressive adult coat. Cords begin forming between the ages of 8 and 12 months, and continue throughout the life of the dog. As new coat grows, the cords will clump together at the base. You will need to spend time every week working on the cords to keep them neat. As you might imagine, it is easy for dirt to get into the cords. If that dirt becomes trapped as the cord tightens, the coat will become discolored and dull looking. The best way to keep a Komondor clean is never to allow it to get dirty. If the dog does get into a mud puddle, then a quick rinse with a garden hose will help get the dirt out."

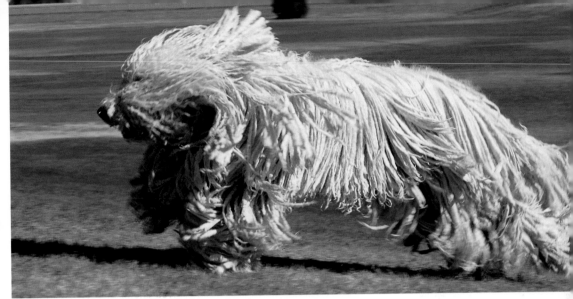

One of the Komondor's most striking features is his corded coat.

Trainability: High, but they are bored by repetition. Needs an experienced, committed owner.

Health Issues: Hip dysplasia, bloat, entropion. Komondorak may be extremely sensitive to some flea and tick products. Like many other stock guard dogs, they are sensitive to anesthesia.

Adoption Option: Komondor Rescue is a non-profit referral organization dedicated to placing unwanted Komondors into new homes. Visit them at www.clubs.akc.org/kca/kca.htm.

Breed Standard in Brief

(Adapted from the Komondor Club of America)

General Appearance: The Komondor is characterized by imposing strength, dignity, courageous demeanor, and pleasing conformation. He is a large, muscular dog with plenty of bone and substance, covered with an unusual, heavy coat of white cords.

Size, Proportion, Substance: Males 27 1/2 inches (70 cm) and up at the withers; females 25 1/2 inches (65 cm) and up at the withers. Dogs are approximately 100 pounds (45 kg) and up, bitches, approximately 80 pounds (36 kg) and up with plenty of bone and substance. While large size is important, type, character, symmetry, movement, and ruggedness are of the greatest importance. The body is slightly longer than the height at the withers.

Head: The head is large. The length of the head from occiput to tip of nose is approximately two-fifths the height of the dog at the withers. The skin around the eyes and on the muzzle is dark.

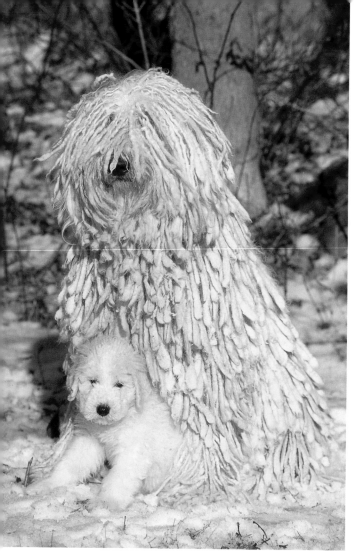

The Komondor has a calm, watchful demeanor.

gated triangle with a slightly rounded tip. They are medium-set and hanging and long enough to reach to the inner corner of the eye on the opposite side of the head. Erect ears or ears that move toward an erect position are a fault. The skull is broad with well-developed arches over the eyes. The occiput is fairly well-developed, and the stop is moderate. The muzzle is wide, coarse, and truncated. Measured from inner corner of the eye to tip of nose the muzzle is two-fifths of the total length of the head. The top of the muzzle is straight and is parallel to the top of the skull. The underjaw is well-developed and broad. Lips are tight and are black in color. Ideally, gums and palate are dark or black. The nose is wide, and the front of the nose forms a right angle with the top of the muzzle. The nostrils are wide. The nose is black. A dark gray or dark brown nose is not desirable but is acceptable. A flesh-colored nose is a disqualification. The bite is scissors; a level bite is acceptable. A distinctly overshot or undershot bite is a fault. Missing teeth are a serious fault. Three or more missing teeth are a disqualification.

The eyes are medium-sized and almond-shaped, not too deeply set. The iris of the eye is dark brown. Edges of the eyelids are gray or black. Light eyes are a fault. Blue eyes are a disqualification. In shape, the ear is an elon-

Neck: The neck is muscular, of medium length, moderately arched, with no dewlap.

Topline: The back is level and strong.

Body: The body is characterized by a powerful, deep chest, which is muscular and proportionately wide. The breast is broad and well-muscled. The belly is somewhat drawn up at the rear. The rump is wide, muscular, and slopes slightly towards the root of the tail. Softness or lack of good muscle tone is a fault.

Tail: The tail is a continuation of the rump line, hanging, and long enough to reach the hocks. Slightly curved upwards and/or to one side at its end. Even when the dog is moving or excited, the greater part of the tail is raised no higher than the level of the back. A short or curly tail is a fault.

Forequarters: Shoulders are well laid back. Forelegs straight, well-boned, and muscular. Viewed from any side, the legs are like vertical columns. The upper arms are carried close to the body.

Feet: The feet are strong, rather large, and with close, well-arched toes. Pads are hard, elastic, and black or gray. Ideally, nails are black or gray.

Hindquarters: The steely, strong bone structure is covered with highly developed muscles. The legs are straight, as viewed from the rear. Stifles are well-bent. Rear dewclaws must be removed.

Coat: Characteristic of the breed is the dense, protective coat. The puppy coat is relatively soft, but it shows a tendency to fall into cord-like curls. The young adult coat, or intermediate coat, consists of very short cords next to the skin, which may be obscured by the sometimes lumpy looking fluff on the outer ends of the cords. The mature coat consists of a dense, soft, woolly undercoat much like the puppy coat, and a coarser outer coat that is wavy or curly. The coarser hairs of the outer coat trap the softer undercoat, forming permanent, strong cords that are felt-like to the touch. A grown dog is entirely covered with a heavy coat of these tassel-like cords, which form naturally. It must be remembered that the length of the Komondor's coat is a function of age, and a younger dog must never be penalized for having a shorter coat. Straight or silky coat is a fault. Failure of the coat to cord by 2 years of age is a disqualification. Short, smooth coat on both head and legs is a disqualification.

Color: Color of the coat is white, but not always the pure white of a brushed coat. A small amount of cream or buff shading is sometimes seen in puppies, but fades with maturity. In the ideal specimen the skin is gray. Pink skin is not desirable but is acceptable. Color other than white, with the exception of small amounts of cream or buff in puppies, is a disqualification.

Gait: The gait is light, leisurely, and balanced. The Komondor takes long strides, is very agile, and light on his feet. The head is carried slightly forward when the dog trots.

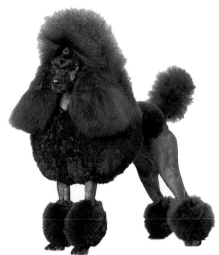

POODLES

Poodles are the classic, or at least most familiar, hypoallergenic dogs. Poodles come in three separate varieties (largest to smallest): Standard, Miniature, and Toy, which compete separately in the show ring, but which have the same standard, except for size. Some people believe the Standard Poodle is the most hypoallergenic of the three, although the Toy obviously sheds less dander because it is the smallest. None of the Poodles have a "doggy" smell. At one time, poodles were used as water retrievers and to find truffles.

Poodles are more intelligent, more dignified, and more sensitive than almost any other breed. They sparkle with personality, and shine with intelligence. By their very nature, Poodles are synonymous with terms like "savoir faire," "joie de vivre," and "insouciance"—in a word,

with everything French. In light of this, it seems kind of too bad that Poodles are probably German. "But they seem so French." Yes, they do, don't they? And in fact, the French have adopted the Poodle as their national dog, of sorts. But the fact is, we're pretty sure that the Poodle, as we know him today, originated in Germany. We even derive the English word "Poodle" from the German *"Pudel,"* which in turn comes from the verb *"Pudelin,"* meaning "to splash around." (Hence "puddle," also.) The word "Poodle" thus means "splasher." This etymology strengthens the theory that the earliest Poodles were water retrievers.

Eventually, the fame of the Poodle spread across Europe, into England, Italy, and Scandinavia. There were Poodles in Belgium and the Netherlands as well, and the Belgians

Supposedly, Belgian Poodles were used to smuggle lace; the animals were shaved, wrapped in lace, and then covered with false hair. I suppose anything is possible with Poodles.

and Dutch apparently thought Poodles were just the thing to hitch up to carts and haul vegetables around with. Luckily, this sort of thing didn't last.

Poodles need daily grooming. The traditional trim was for practical reasons: leaving the hair long to protect the heart and chest from cold water, and clipping the legs to decrease drag while swimming. Later, the French added the pompons and ribbons that are seen in the show ring today.

Vital Statistics

National Breed Club: Poodle Club of America. Visit them at www.poodleclubofamerica.org/usamap.htm.

Origin: Europe, either Germany or Russia. Today, however, it is the national dog of France.

Group: Toy (Toy Poodle); Non-sporting (Standard and Miniature) (AKC)/Utility Group (KC).

Size: The Poodles comes in three sizes:
Standard: Over 15 inches (38 cm) at the shoulder.
Miniature: Between 10 and 15 inches (25 and 38 cm) at the shoulder.

Toy: Under 10 inches (38 cm) at the shoulder.

Lifespan: 13 to 15 years. Smaller Poodles live longest.

Colors: Any solid color including white, black, silver, blue, apricot, or brown.

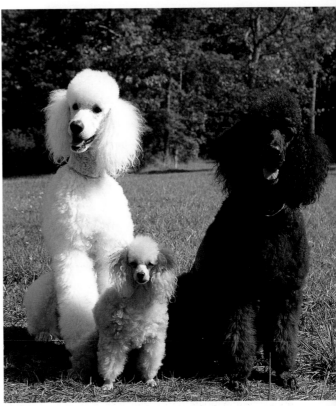

Poodles come in three sizes: Toy, Miniature and Standard

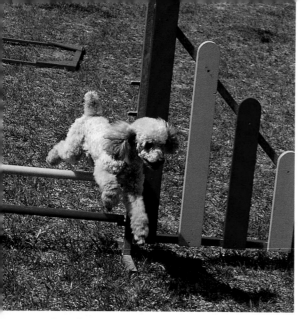

Poodles are easily trained and enjoy activities like agility.

Grooming: Single, harsh, curly coat. All varieties need daily grooming and regular clipping. Professional grooming is recommended for a show-like coat, but many people learn a simple clip to do themselves. Only certain clips are permitted in the show ring; if your Poodle is a pet, you can suit your fancy by creating a coat of original design or keep it closely trimmed for utmost allergenic effect.

Personality: Friendly, proud, intuitive.

Sociability: Superior family dog; may be reserved around strangers. Excellent with children, especially the Standard. Enjoys the company of other Poodles. Poodles enjoy being treated as members of the family.

Activity Level: Medium to High.

Trainability: Extremely High.

Health Issues: Addison's disease, progressive retinal atrophy (Miniature and Toy), optic nerve hypoplasia (Standard), distichiasis, Legg-Perthes (Miniature and Toy), glaucoma, luxating patella (Toy and Miniature), cancer, epilepsy (Toy and Miniature), sebaceous adenitis (Standard), ear infections, conjunctivitis, enteritis, entropion, cardiomyopathy (Standard), mitral valve insufficiency (Toy and Miniature), hip dysplasia (Standard and Miniature), hypothyroidism, allergies, bloat (Standard).

Adoption Option: For information about Poodle Rescue, visit the Poodle Club of America at www.poodleclubofamerica.org and click on Rescue.

Breed Standard in Brief

(Adapted from the Poodle Club of America)

General Appearance, Carriage, and Condition: The Poodle is active and elegant. He is squarely built and well-proportioned.

Size, Proportion, Substance: The Standard Poodle is over 15 inches (38 cm) at the highest point of the shoulders. Any Poodle that is 15 inches (38 cm) or less in height shall be disqualified from competition as a Standard Poodle. The Miniature Poodle is 15 inches (38 cm) or under at the highest point of the shoulders, with a minimum height in excess of 10 inches (25 cm). Any Poodle that is over

15 inches (38 cm) or is 10 inches (25 cm) or less at the highest point of the shoulders shall be disqualified from competition as a Miniature Poodle. The Toy Poodle is 10 inches (25 cm) or under at the highest point of the shoulders. Any Poodle that is more than 10 inches (25 cm) at the highest point of the shoulders shall be disqualified from competition as a Toy Poodle. To be in proportion, the length of body measured from the breastbone to the point of the rump approximates the height from the highest point of the shoulders to the ground. The bone and muscle of both forelegs and hind legs are in proportion to size of dog.

Head and Expression: The eyes are very dark, oval, and set far enough apart and positioned to create an alert, intelligent expression. Round, protruding, large, or very light eyes are a major fault. The ears should hang close to the head, set at or slightly below eye level. The ear leather is long, wide and thickly feathered; however, the ear fringe should not be of excessive length. The skull is moderately rounded, with a slight but definite stop. Cheekbones and muscles are flat. Length from occiput to stop is about the same as the length of muzzle. The muzzle is long, straight, and fine, with slight chiseling under the eyes. The chin should be definite enough to preclude snipiness. Lack of chin is a major fault. The teeth are white, strong, and

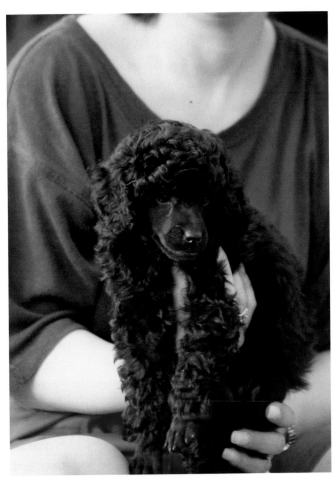

Poodles can make excellent family dogs.

with a scissors bite. Undershot, overshot, or wry mouth is a major fault.

Neck, Topline, Body: The neck is well proportioned, strong, and long enough to permit the head to be carried high and with dignity. Skin should be snug at the throat. The neck rises from strong, smoothly muscled shoulders. A ewe neck is a major fault. The topline is level, with the exception of a slight hollow just behind the shoulder. The chest is deep and moderately wide, with well sprung ribs. The loin is short, broad, and muscular. The tail is straight, set on high and carried up, docked enough to ensure a balanced outline. A tail set low, curled, or carried over the back is a major fault.

Forequarters: The shoulders are strong and smoothly muscled. The shoulder blade is well laid back and about the same length as the upper foreleg. A steep shoulder is a major fault. The forelegs are straight and parallel when viewed from the front. When viewed from the side, the elbow is directly below the highest point of the shoulder. The pasterns are strong. Dewclaws may be removed. The feet are rather small, and oval. The toes are well arched and cushioned on thick firm pads. Nails short but not to excess. The feet turn neither in nor out. A paper or splay foot is a major fault.

Hindquarters: The angulation of the hindquarters balances that of the forequarters. The hind legs are straight and parallel when viewed from the rear. They are muscular and wide in the region of the stifles, which are well bent. The femur and tibia are about equal in length; hock to heel is short and perpendicular to the ground. When standing, the rear toes are only slightly behind the point of the rump. Cow hocks are a major fault.

Coat: The coat is dense, with a harsh texture. It may be kept in curls or corded. In either case, the standard calls for the coat to be of varying length for show. A show coat is longer on the mane or body coat, head, and ears; it is shorter on puffs, bracelets, and pompons. Special clips are mandated for show poodles also.

Color: The coat is an even and solid color at the skin. In blues, grays, silvers, browns, cafe-au-laits, apricots, and creams the coat may show varying shades of the same color. Clear colors are preferred. Parti-colored dogs are disqualified.

Gait: The poodle moves in a straightforward trot, with light springy action and strong hindquarters drive. Head and tail carried up. Sound, effortless movement is essential.

Temperament: Carrying himself proudly, very active, intelligent, the Poodle has about him an air of distinction and dignity peculiar to himself. Shyness or sharpness is a major fault.

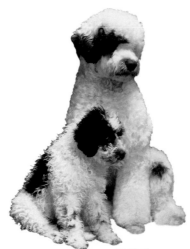

PORTUGUESE WATER DOG

The Portuguese Water Dog (PWD) was developed by fishermen along the coasts of Portugal, although a minority report suggests that the Goths first created the breed. Its job was to herd fish into the nets, to retrieve lost tackle, and to act as a messenger from ship to ship, or ship to shore. They were also employed as "barkers" on foggy days to keep ships from colliding with each other

The Portuguese Water Dog is a calm dog of excellent temperament. These are wonderful dogs for water work.

For the allergy sufferer, the PWD has the advantage of not only a curly, low-shedding coat, but also a single rather than a double coat, which means there is less hair to fly around the house.

In Portugal, the breed is called Cao de Agua (pronounced Kown-d'Ahgwa), which also means water dog.

Vital Statistics

National Club: Portuguese Water Dog Club of America. Visit them at www.pwdca.org.

Origin: Portugal during the Middle Ages.

Group: Working Group (KC and AKC).

Size: 17 to 23 inches (43 to 58 cm); 35 to 60 pounds (16 to 27 kg).

Lifespan: 9 to 15 years.

Colors: Solid black, brown, white, particolor.

Grooming: Needs frequent brushing and professional grooming every 6 to 8 weeks. They

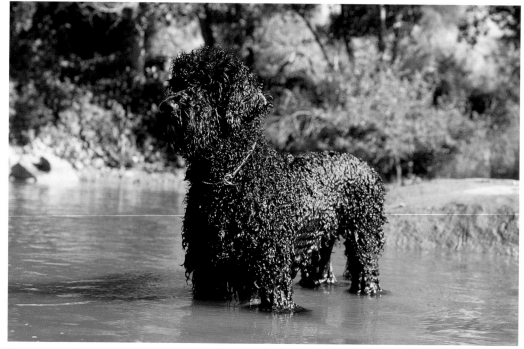
Portuguese Water Dogs are wonderful dogs for water work.

can be clipped in the lion clip (which leaves a naked behind) or in the more modest retriever clip.

Personality: Active, bouncy, brave, willful.

Sociability: Tends to bond to one person. More reserved with others. Generally OK with other pets, although he can be jealous.

Activity Level: High; however they are comfortable in a small apartment.

Trainability: High.

Health Issues: Orthopedic problems (hip dysplasia), Addison's disease, glycogen storage disease (GM1), eye problems (progressive reti-

nal atrophy).

Adoption Option: The primary responsibility of the Portuguese Water Dog Rescue & Relocation Program is to help all PWDs who are in need of a new home. Visit them at www.pwdca.org/rescue.html.

Breed Standard in Brief

(Adapted from Portuguese Water Dog Club of America)

General Appearance: This dog has a robust, medium build, with two possible coat types: curly and wavy. He has an impressive head of considerable breadth and well-proportioned mass, a rugged body, and a powerful, thick-based tail, carried gallantly.

Size, Proportion, Substance: Males range from 20 to 23 inches (51 to 58 cm) at the withers, with the ideal at 22 inches (56 cm). Females range from 17 to 21 inches (43 to 53 cm), with the ideal at 19 inches (48 cm). Males weigh 42 to 60 pounds (19 to 27 kg); females, 35 to 50 pounds (16 to 23 kg). The PWD is slightly longer than tall when measured from prosternum to rearmost point of the buttocks, and from withers to ground. He has strong, substantial bone; well developed, neither refined nor coarse, and a solidly built, muscular body. Lack of substance or muscle is a major fault.

Head: The head is one of the most important features of the PWD. It should be distinctively large, well proportioned, and with exceptional breadth of topskull. A small, narrow, unimpressive head is a major fault. His expression is steady, penetrating, and attentive. The eyes are medium in size; roundish, set well apart, and a bit obliquely. They are neither prominent nor sunken. Black or various tones of brown in color, but darker eyes are preferred. Eye rims should fully pigmented with black edges in black, black-and-white, or white dogs; brown edges in brown dogs. The ears should set well above the line of the eye. Leather is heart-shaped and thin. Except for a small open-ing at the back, ears are held nicely against the head. Tips should not reach below the lower jaw. The skull is slightly longer than the muzzle in profile, its curvature more accentuated at the back than in the front. When viewed head-on, the top of the skull is very broad and appears domed, with a slight depression in the middle. The forehead is prominent, and has a central furrow, extending two-thirds of the distance from stop to a well-defined occiput. The stop is well defined. The muzzle is substantial, and wider at the base than at the nose. A snipey muzzle is a major fault. The nose is broad with flared nostrils. It is fully pigmented; black in

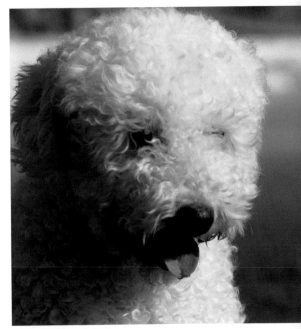

The head is one of the most important features of the Portuguese Water Dog.

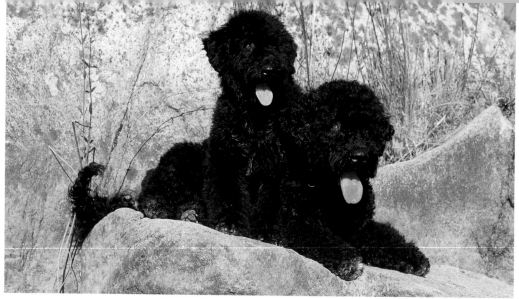

The Portuguese Water Dog has no undercoat.

dogs with black, black-and-white, or white coats; various tones of brown in dogs with brown coats. The lips are thick, especially in front; no flew. Lips and mucous membranes are quite black, or well ticked with black in dogs with black, black-and-white, or white coats; various tones of brown in dogs with brown coats. The bite is scissors or level. Overshot or undershot bite is a major fault.

Neck, Topline, Body: The neck is straight, short, round, and held high. It is strongly muscled with no dewlap. The topline is level and firm. The chest is broad and deep, reaching down to the elbow. Ribs are long and well-sprung. The abdomen is well held up in a graceful line. The back is broad and well muscled. The loin is short and meets the croup smoothly. The croup is well formed and only slightly inclined,

with hip bones hardly apparent. The tail is undocked; thick at the base and tapering; set slightly below the line of the back; it should not reach below the hock. When the dog is attentive, the tail is held in a ring, the front of which should not reach forward of the loin.

Forequarters: The shoulders are well inclined and very strongly muscled. The forelegs are strong and straight, with long, well-muscled forearms. The knee is heavy-boned, wider in front than at the side. Pasterns are long and strong. Dewclaws may be removed. Feet are round and rather flat. Webbing between the toes is of soft skin, well covered with hair, and reaches the toe tips. Central pad is very thick, others normal. Nails held up slightly off the ground. Black, brown, white, and striped nails are allowed.

Hindquarters: The hindquarters are powerful and well-balanced with the front. The legs, viewed from the rear, are parallel to each other, straight and strongly muscled. No dewclaws. Feet as in forefeet.

Coat: The coat is thick and profuse, covering the whole body evenly, except where the forearm meets the brisket and in the groin area, where it is thinner. No undercoat, mane, or ruff. Sparse, wispy, brittle, wiry, naturally short, close-lying hair, partially or over all is a major fault. A double coat is also a major fault. There are two varieties of coat: curly and wavy. The curly coat is compact, cylindrical curls, somewhat lusterless. The hair on the ears is sometimes wavy. The wavy coat falls gently in waves, not curls, and with a slight sheen. For the show ring, two clips are acceptable: the lion and retriever clips. In the lion clip, as soon as the coat grows long, the middle part and hindquarters, as well as the muzzle, are clipped. The hair at the end of the tail is left at full length. In the retriever clip, in order to give a natural appearance and a smooth unbroken line, the entire coat is scissored or clipped to follow the outline of the dog, leaving a short blanket of coat no longer than 1 inch in length. The hair at the end of the tail is left at full length.

Color: Black, white, and various tones of brown; also combinations of black or brown with white. A white coat does not imply albinism provided nose, mouth, and eyelids are black. In animals with black, white, or black-and-white coats, the skin is decidedly bluish.

Gait: Short, lively steps when walking. The trot is a forward striding, well-balanced movement.

Temperament: An animal of spirited disposition, self-willed, brave, and very resistant to fatigue. A dog of exceptional intelligence and a loyal companion, it obeys its master with facility and apparent pleasure. It is obedient with those who look after it or with those for whom it works. Shy, vicious, or unsound behavior is a major fault.

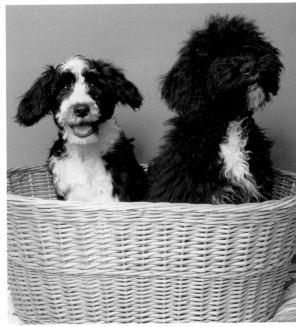

PWDs come in various combinations of black and white.

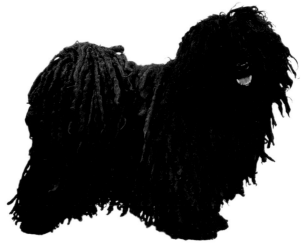

PULI

Like the other Hungarian sheepdog in this book, the Komondor, the Puli may have come to Hungary from Central Asia with the Magyar people. Some experts believe the breed can be traced back to as early as 4500 B.C. It is said that a good Puli was worth a year's salary to a shepherd. Granted, shepherds probably didn't make very much, but there you are.

The Puli coat can be either wavy or curly. If left to grow out, it will form "cords," which begin to develop when the puppy is about 9 months old, but which may not mature until the dog is 5 years old.

If you enter your Puli in obedience or agility, you can tie the hair away from its eyes, although Puli enthusiasts claim that the dog can see perfectly through his curtain of hair. Puli also excel in herding, which is a great event to participate in, unless you are allergic to wool!

The plural of Puli is Pulik. Oh, by the way, Hungary makes a car called the Puli, too.

Vital Statistics

National Breed Club: Puli Club of America. Visit them at www.puli-club.org.

Origin: Hungary during the Middle Ages.

Group: Herding (AKC)/Pastoral Group (KC).

Size: 15 to 18 inches (38 to 46 cm); 29 to 33 pounds (12 to 15 kg).

Lifespan: 11 to 16 years.

Colors: Rusty black, dull black, black, white, gray, apricot.

Grooming: Ground-length corded, weather-resistant coat. The outer coat wavy but not silky, the undercoat soft, woolly, dense. Very high maintenance. A heavily coated Puli can take up to an hour to bathe and may take up to 3 days to air dry and 6 hours or more to dry with the use of a blow dryer. You have to get the dog dry or else he could mildew (really). The owner must keep an eye on the cords to make sure they are open to the skin.

Personality: Energetic, devoted, affectionate.

Sociability: Tends to be a one-person or family dog. Not especially good with children, aloof to stranger, many be aggressive to other breeds (likes other Pulik).

Activity Level: Very High.

Trainability: Medium.

Health Issues: Eye problems, hearing problems, hip dysplasia.

Adoption Option: Luckily for Pulik, few are available through rescue, although you may get lucky. For more information, go to www.puliclub.org/PCARescue.htm.

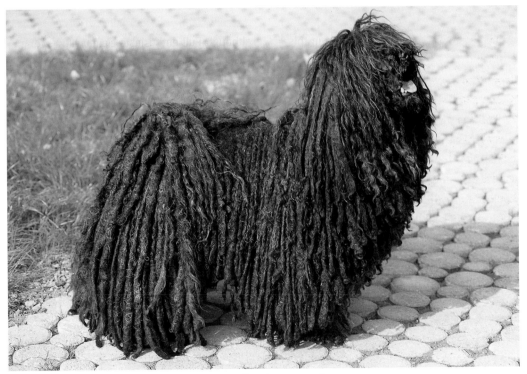

Striking and highly characteristic is the Puli's shaggy coat.

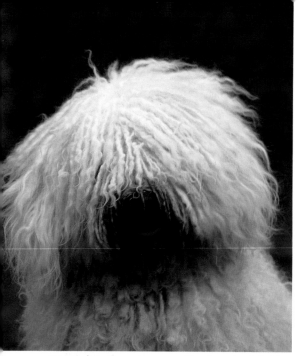

The Puli is by nature an affectionate, intelligent, and home-loving companion.

Breed Standard in Brief

(Adapted from the Puli Club of America)

General Appearance: The Puli is a compact, square appearing, well-balanced dog of medium size. Striking and highly characteristic is the shaggy coat.

Size, Proportion, Substance: Ideally, males are 17 inches (43 cm) measured from the withers to the ground; females, 16 inches (41 cm). An inch over or under these measurements is acceptable. The tightly knit body approximates a square measured from withers to ground and point of shoulder to point of buttock. Medium bone.

Head: The head is of medium size. The almond-shaped eyes are deep set, rather large, and dark brown with black or slate-gray eye rims. The medium size, V-shaped ears, set on somewhat higher than the level of the eyes, are hanging, about half the head length. The skull slightly domed and medium broad. The stop is defined, but not abrupt. The muzzle is strong and straight, a third of the head length, and ends in a nose of good size. The nose is always black. Flews and gums are black or slate gray. A full complement of teeth, comparatively large, that meet in a scissors bite.

Neck, Topline, Body: The neck is strong and free of throatiness. The back is level and strong, of medium length, with croup sloping slightly. The chest is moderately broad and deep; the ribs are well sprung. The loin is short, strong, and moderately tucked up. The tail is carried over, and blends into the backline.

Forequarters: The shoulders are well laid back. Upper arm and scapula are approximately equal in length and form an angle of 90 degrees. The forelegs are straight, strong, and medium boned, with strong and flexible pasterns. Dewclaws may be removed. The round, compact feet have well arched toes and thick cushioned pads. The pads and nails are black or slate gray.

Hindquarters: The hindquarters are well developed and muscular with well bent stifles, the rear assembly balancing that of the front.

The hocks are perpendicular to the ground and well let down. Dewclaws, if any, may be removed. Feet as in front.

Coat: The dense, weather resistant coat is profuse on all parts of the body. The outer coat is wavy or curly, but never silky. The undercoat is soft, wooly, and dense. The coat clumps together easily and, if allowed to develop naturally, will form cords in the adult. The cords are wooly, varying in shape and thickness, either flat or round, depending on the texture of the coat and the balance of undercoat to outer coat. The Puli may be shown either corded or brushed. It is essential that the proper double coat with correct texture always be apparent. With age, the coat can become quite long, even reaching to the ground; however, only enough length to properly evaluate quality and texture is considered necessary so as not to penalize the younger or working specimens.

Color: Only the solid colors of rusty black, black, all shades of gray, and white are acceptable; however, on the chest, a white spot of not more than 2 inches is permissible. In the black and the gray dogs, an intermixture of some gray, black, or white hairs is acceptable as long as the overall appearance of a solid color is maintained. The fully pigmented skin has a bluish or gray cast whatever the coat color.

Gait: The Puli is typically a lively, acrobatic dog; light, quick, agile, and able to change directions instantly. At a collected or contained trot, the gait is distinctive: quick-stepping and animated, not far reaching, yet in no way mincing or stilted. When at a full trot, the Puli covers ground smoothly and efficiently, with good reach and drive.

Temperament: By nature an affectionate, intelligent, and home-loving companion, the Puli is sensibly suspicious and therefore an excellent watchdog. Extreme timidity is a serious fault.

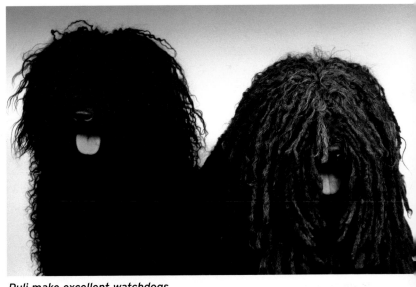

Puli make excellent watchdogs.

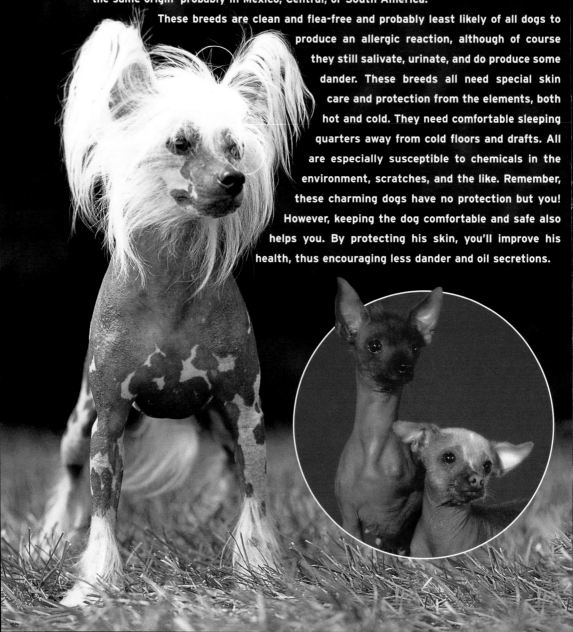

PART 2
HAIRLESS BREEDS

It is believed that, with the exception of the American Hairless Terrier, all hairless breeds have the same origin—probably in Mexico, Central, or South America.

These breeds are clean and flea-free and probably least likely of all dogs to produce an allergic reaction, although of course they still salivate, urinate, and do produce some dander. These breeds all need special skin care and protection from the elements, both hot and cold. They need comfortable sleeping quarters away from cold floors and drafts. All are especially susceptible to chemicals in the environment, scratches, and the like. Remember, these charming dogs have no protection but you! However, keeping the dog comfortable and safe also helps you. By protecting his skin, you'll improve his health, thus encouraging less dander and oil secretions.

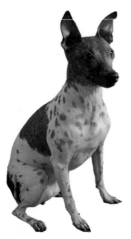

AMERICAN HAIRLESS TERRIER
(HAIRLESS VARIETY)

This is my number one pick for people with dog allergies. Many people who cannot tolerate any other breed of dog can live happily with an American Hairless Terrier (AHT). While other hairless breeds do have some hair on the head, feet, or tail, the AHT is truly almost hairless. In addition, AHTs have full dentition (arrangement of teeth), whereas the other hairless breeds tend to have both missing or weak teeth. The AHT is also notably free of skin problems.

The first American Hairless Terrier (Josephine) was born in Louisiana, during the fall of 1972, in a litter of Rat Terriers. Josephine had silky skin, black spots—and no hair. Josephine was a charming, bright, loyal dog who won hearts everywhere. It was obvi-

ous there should be more just like her!

The breeders were Willie and Edwin Scott, and they sought from the outset to make the American Hairless Terrier a separate breed, working with both a geneticist and a veterinarian. They eventually named their establishment Trout Creek Kennel. Although a new breed was their goal, at first, the Scotts and other breeders agreed for the time being to allow the dogs to enter the UKC registry as "Rat Terriers, hairless variety." (The Rat Terrier was recognized by the United Kennel Club in 1999.) In 2004, the United Kennel Club recognized the AHT as a separate breed. The parent breed, the Rat Terrier, is being evaluated for AKC recognition.

AHT puppies are born with a soft, vestigi-

AHTs are themselves subject to several kinds of allergies, most commonly grass allergies, which gives them a rash.

al "down" that generally covers the body. This down gradually diminishes, until age 6 to 8 weeks, by which time the pup should be completely hairless, except for whiskers and eyebrows. The shed begins at the head and proceeds towards the rear.

Their skin, typically pink with spots of black, gray, brown, or red, but which can be lemon or even blue, is soft to the touch. The AHT does not shed hair, but like any other mammal, it does shed skin cells—in this case about every 20 days, so there is a little (very little) dander.

However, these dogs need careful protec-

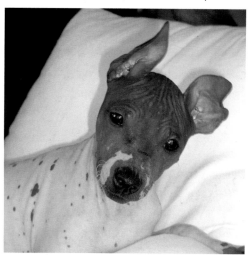

The skin of the AHT is typically pink with spots of black, gray, brown, or red, and is soft to the touch.

tion from the sun and sweaters when it gets cold. They need sun block or even T-shirts if they are outside. Because these courageous dogs lack a protective coat, they are extremely prone to cuts and scratches as they charge through the bushes and the like. They need to be carefully and frequently checked for injuries.

Believe it or not, members of this breed will actually break out in a sweat when they are hot or frightened. They can also get pimples, although they are free from many of the other skin diseases that plague hairless dogs. They are also free of the breeding problems we see in other hairless breeds. These dogs almost never drool! (They need to conserve their heat.)

This breed retains a strong hunting instinct and needs to be watched carefully around tiny pets. He is an excellent family dog or companion to the elderly. This breed does well in apartments if given opportunity to exercise.

One wonderful thing about owners of the AHTs is that they are willing to assist you in allergy testing! Visit the American Hairless Terrier Association for a list of families who are willing to help you "allergy test" to see if an AHT is right for you! Volunteers are scattered throughout the United States, Canada, and Northern Europe.

Vital Statistics

National Breed Club: American Hairless Terrier Association. Visit them at www.ahta.info.

Origin: United States (1972).

Group: Terrier (UKC).

Size: The breed comes in two sizes:

> Toy: 7.5 to 11 inches (19 to 28 cm); 4 to 8 pounds. (2 to 4 kg).
>
> Miniature: 11.5 to 16 inches (29 to 41 cm); 8.5 to 16 pounds (4 to 7 kg).

Lifespan: 12 to 16 years.

Colors: All colors accepted, but skin is usually spotted or parti-colored. The spots enlarge with age and darken in the sun.

Grooming: Skin protection, such as sun block during the summer and lotion with or without lanolin in dry weather. Can be bathed several times a week with no ill effects.

Personality: Friendly, tenacious, lively, intelligent.

Sociability: Good with well-behaved children, other dogs, family cats; may attack mice.

Activity Level: High.

Trainability: High.

Health Issues: Luxating patella (slipping kneecap); Legg-Calve-Perthes disease (deterioration of the hip ball joint). The AHT Association maintains a health and genetic screening database to collect information about the breed and prevent genetic health problems.

Adoption Option: For information on American Hairless Terrier Rescue, go to www.ahta.info/rtrescue.html.

Breed Standard in Brief

(Adapted from American Hairless Terrier Association)

Since the American Hairless Terrier is directly descended from the Rat Terrier, he is identical in build and character. This is an active, small-to-medium terrier. The preferred ratio of length of body (point of chest to point of buttocks) to height at withers is 10:9. The head is broad, slightly domed, wedge-shaped, and proportionate to the size of the body. The ears are V-shaped, set at the outside edges of the skull, and can be erect, tipped, or button. He carries his tail in an upward curve. (The coated variety may have a docked tail for show purposes, the hairless never.)

Head: The head is proportionate to the size of the body. When viewed from the side, the skull and muzzle are of equal length and joined by a moderate (not abrupt) stop. Viewed from the front and the side, the American Hairless Terrier's head forms a blunt wedge. The skull is broad and slightly domed, tapering slightly toward the muzzle. The jaws are powerful, with well-muscled cheeks. An "apple-shaped" skull is a fault. The muzzle is well filled-out under the eyes,

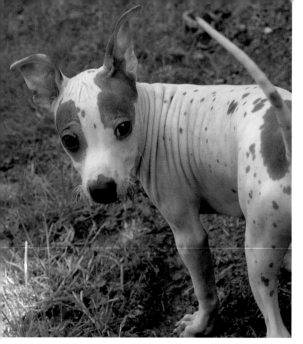

American Hairless Terriers are friendly, tenacious, lively, and intelligent.

spotted) nose is a fault. The eyes are set obliquely and are round, of moderate size, and somewhat prominent. Eye rims match nose pigment. Eye color ranges from dark brown to amber and corresponds with skin color. Hazel eyes are acceptable in dogs with lighter skin color. Blue or amber eyes are permitted in blue-colored dogs only, but a dark gray eye with gray eye rims is preferred. Bulgy or deep-set eyes; light-colored eyes in a dog with black pigment; eyes not of matching colors; eye with iris containing more than one color; wall or china eye are faults. The ears are V-shaped, set at the outside edges of the skull. Erect ears are preferred, but tipped or button ears are acceptable. Hanging ears are a disqualification. Matching ears are strongly preferred. Nonmatching ear carriage should be penalized to the degree of the variation. Note: Ear carriage may not stabilize until a dog is mature. Dogs under 1 year of age should not be penalized for variations in ear carriage. Erect ears, with the sides curved inward forming a tulip shape; rose ears; flying ears; nonmatching ear carriages are faults.

well-chiseled, and tapering slightly from the stop to the nose. Jaws are powerful and hinged well back, allowing the dog to open his mouth wide enough to catch rats and other rodents. Lips are dry and tight with no flews. Lip pigment matches nose pigment. A "snipey" muzzle is a fault. Teeth must be complete, white, evenly spaced, and of a good size. (Many of the other hairless breeds have missing premolars or other dentition.) A scissors bite is preferred, but a level bite is acceptable. Missing teeth and undershot or overshot bite is a fault. The nose is black or self-colored (same color as coat). A Dudley (liver) or butterfly (partially pigmented or

Neck: The neck is clean, moderately long, smoothly muscled, slightly arched, and tapers slightly from the shoulders to the head. The neck blends smoothly into well laid back shoulders.

Forequarters: The shoulders are smoothly

muscled. The shoulder blades are well laid back with the upper tips fairly close together at the withers. The upper arm appears to be equal in length to the shoulder blade and joins it at an apparent right angle. The elbows are close to the body. Viewed from any angle, the forelegs are straight, strong, and sturdy in bone. The pasterns are strong, short, and nearly vertical.

Hindquarters: The hindquarters are muscular, with the length of the upper and lower thighs being about equal. The angulation of the hindquarters is in balance with the angulation of the forequarters. The stifles are well-bent, and the hocks are well let down. When the dog is standing, the short, strong rear pasterns are perpendicular to the ground and, viewed from the rear, parallel to one another.

Feet: The feet are compact and slightly oval in shape. The two middle toes are slightly longer than the other toes. Toes may be well split up but not flat or splayed. Front dewclaws may be removed. Rear dewclaws must be removed. Flat feet, splayed feet, and rear dewclaws are faults.

Tail: The tail is thick at the base and tapers toward the tip. When the dog is alert, the tail is carried in an upward curve. When relaxed, the tail may be carried straight out behind the dog. Bent or ring tails are faults. Natural bobtail is a disqualification.

Skin/Coat: A mature American Hairless Terrier, Hairless variety, is free from hair except for whiskers and guard hairs on the muzzle, and eyebrows. Short, very fine (vellus) hair may be present on the body of a mature dog. The skin is smooth and warm to the touch. Vellus hair (down) longer than 1 mm on a dog over 6 months of age is a serious fault.

Color: Any skin color is acceptable. The skin is usually parti-colored with an underlying skin color and freckles or spots of contrasting color. Freckles enlarge with age, and skin color will darken when exposed to the sun. Albinism is a fault.

Gait: The American Hairless Terrier moves with a jaunty air that suggests agility, speed, and power. American Hairless Terrier gait is smooth and effortless, with good reach of forequarters without any trace of hackney gait. Rear quarters have strong driving power, with hocks fully extending. Viewed from any position, legs turn neither in nor out, nor do feet cross or interfere with each other. As speed increases, feet tend to converge toward center line of balance.

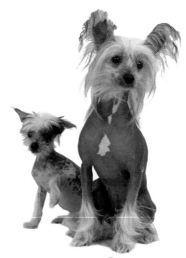

CHINESE CRESTED
(HAIRLESS TYPE)

Most experts believe the Chinese Crested originated South and Central America, not China. The dogs turned out to be superior ratters, although one would think their lack of fur made them vulnerable to biting. (If you do decide on a Chinese Crested and have rats in the house, an exterminator would be a better bet.) A rival theory suggests the origin of the breed is Africa, and the Chinese knew them as "African Terriers." However, it is not completely clear that ancient navigators knew Africa from South America. (Columbus was certainly confused—he thought Cuba was India.)

Chinese Cresteds come in two varieties: the Hairless and the Powderpuff or coated variety. The Hairless has hair only on the head, tail, and feet. Both varieties are born in the same litter. They are shown together in the conformation ring, and are judged by the same standard, except for the coat, making allowance for incomplete definition in the hairless variety. Only the hairless variety is hypoallergenic.

They will need a sweater in the winter, but (and you should sympathize) many of them are allergenic to wool or lanolin! Choose the fabric carefully.

Like many other hairless breeds, some Chinese Cresteds have an incomplete set of teeth, so chewing bones is difficult for them. They are also inclined to obesity.

The Chinese Crested makes a great companion dog, but cannot tolerate the cold.

The most famous breeder of Chinese Cresteds was Gypsy Rose Lee, the stripper. The moral, I suppose, is that there is an innate connection between naked dogs and naked ladies.

Vital Statistics

National Breed Club: American Chinese Crested Club. Visit them at www.chinesecrestedclub.info.

Origin: Possibly Central or South America, then taken to China and port cities where Chinese ships were trading. Known in Europe in 1500s, but undoubtedly bred much earlier.

Group: Toy (AKC and KC).

Size: 9 to 13 inches (23 to 33 cm); 11 to 13 pounds (5 to 6 kg).

Lifespan: 13 to 15 years.

Colors: Any color or combination of colors acceptable.

Grooming: Need sunscreen when outdoors in the summer.

Personality: Happy, affectionate, playful, devoted, cheerful.

Sociability: Excellent with children and other pets.

Activity Level: Medium.

Trainability: Medium to High, requires gentle handling.

Health Issues: Legg-Perthes, skin problems, infections.

Adoption Option: Crest-Care, Inc., whose goals are to preserve and protect Chinese Cresteds in need. Visit them at www.crest-care.com.

Breed Standard in Brief

(Adapted from American Chinese Crested Club)

General Appearance: Fine-boned and graceful.

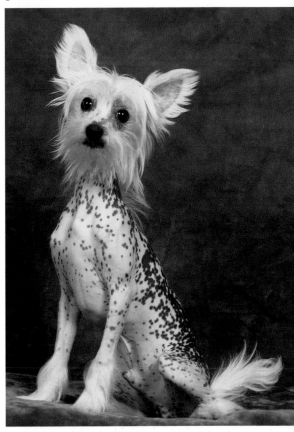

The Chinese Crested makes a great companion dog, but cannot tolerate the cold.

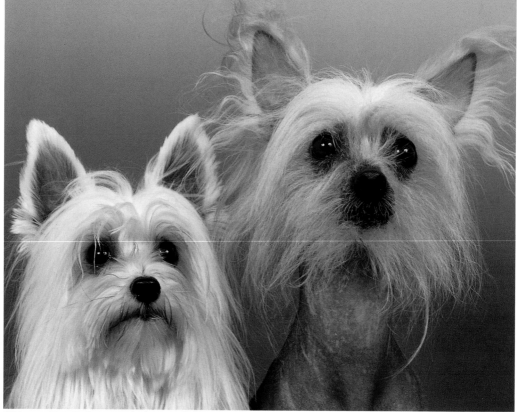

Chinese Cresteds come in two varieties: Hairless and Powderpuff.

Size, Proportion, Substance: The ideal size is 11 to 13 inches (28 to 33 cm), but larger or smaller dogs are not faulty. The body is rectangular in shape, and slender without appearing fragile.

Head: The Chinese Crested has an alert expression, with almond-shaped eyes set wide apart. Darker dogs have darker eyes. The eye rims should match the dog's coloring. The ears are uncropped. Large, and erect, set so that the base of the ear is level with the outside corner of the eye. The skull is arched gently.

The distance from occiput to the slight but distinct stop is equal to the distance from stop to tip of nose. The head is wedge-shaped. The cheeks taper cleanly into the muzzle. The nose is dark in dark-colored dogs, but may be lighter in lighter-colored dogs. The nose pigment is solid. The lips are clean and tight. A scissors or level bite is expected. The Hairless variety is not to be penalized for absence of full dentition.

Neck, Topline, Body: The neck is lean and clean, slightly arched, and carried high. The topline is level to the slightly sloping croup. The brisket extends to the elbow. The breastbone is not prominent. Ribs are well developed. The depth of the chest tapers to a moderate tuck-up at the flanks. The tail is slender and tapers to a curve. It is long enough to reach the hock and is carried gaily when the dog is in motion. It may be carried slightly forward over the back. At rest, the tail is down with a slight curve upward at the end. Two-thirds of the end of the tail is covered by long, flowing feathering, referred to as a *plume.*

Forequarters: The angulation or layback of the shoulders is 45 degrees. The shoulders are clean and narrow. The elbows are close to body, and the legs are long, slender, and straight. The pasterns are upright, fine, and strong. Dewclaws may be removed. The Chinese Crested has a hare foot, narrow with elongated toes. Nails are trimmed to moderate length.

Hindquarters: The stifle is moderately angulated, but perpendicular from hock joint to ground. Dewclaws may be removed. The feet are the same as for forequarters.

Coat: The Hairless variety has hair on certain portions of the body: the head (called a *crest*), the tail (called a *plume*), and the feet from the toes to the front pasterns and rear hock joints (called *socks*). The texture of all hair is soft and silky, flowing to any length. Placement of hair is not as important as overall type. Wherever the body is hairless, the skin is soft and smooth. Head Crest begins at the stop and tapers off between the base of the skull and the back of the neck. Hair on the ears and face is permitted on the Hairless and may be trimmed for neatness. Tail plume is described under tail.

Color: Any color or combination of colors.
Gait: Lively, agile, and smooth without being stilted or hackneyed.

Temperament: Gay and alert.

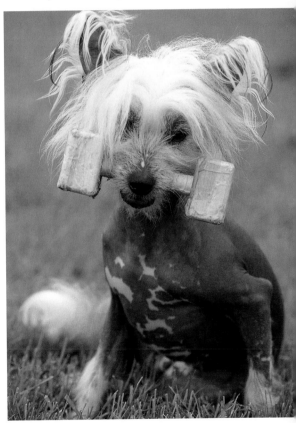

Chinese Cresteds are gay and alert little dogs.

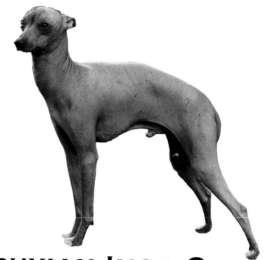

PERUVIAN INCA ORCHID/ PERUVIAN HAIRLESS

It is suggested that this breed was developed by the Moche people of Peru, before or during the eighth century. In the ancient Peruvian language of Quechua they were called "Ca-Allepo," which means "dogs without garments." The Spanish named them "Perros Flora" or "flower dogs" and, in the United States and parts of Europe, they are called Peruvian Inca Orchid or simply Perro Sin Pello del Peru (Peruvian dogs without hair). Like other hairless breeds, however, the Peruvian comes in both coated and hairless varieties. The hairless variety produces fewer allergens.

The Inca believed these dogs were gifts from the gods and thought them to have healing capabilities. They had good sense about this breed, however, and never allowed them to roam free, except at night. Apparently, they saw first-hand what sunburn could do to a hairless dog.

The breed is really a sighthound, and has a strong prey drive. Socialization as a puppy is very important! One of the most notable characteristics of the breed is the "kissing spot" on the top of the head.

> Many hairless breeds also lack teeth. There's a stronger connection between teeth and hair that you might think.

Vital Statistics

National Club: Peruvian Inca Orchid Dog Club

of America. Visit them at www.willabe.com/index.html.

Origin: Peru.

Group: Hound (AKC)/Toy (other registries).

Size: 20 to 23 inches (51 to 58 cm); 30 to 40 pounds (14 to 18 kg).

Lifespan: 12 to 15 years.

Colors: Any color accepted, but most are black with pink spots.

Grooming: Skin care. They need protection from direct sun and cold.

Personality: Calm, independent. Reserved with strangers.

Sociability: Needs early socialization.

Activity Level: Low.

Trainability: Medium.

Health Issues: Very few.

Breed Standard in Brief

(Adapted from Peruvian Inca Orchid Club of America)

General Appearance: A slender sighthound of moderate size with an elegant, fit appearance.

Temperament: Adult dogs will be calm and quiet, but reserved with strangers. Highly

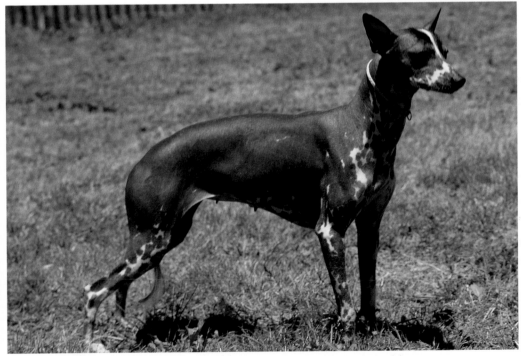

The Peruvian Inca Orchid is really a sighthound, and has a strong prey drive.

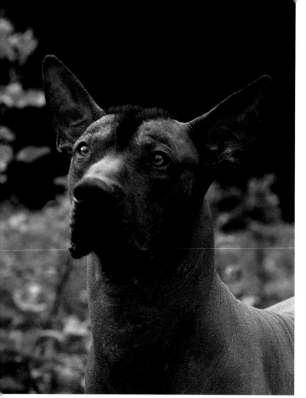

One of the most notable characteristics of the breed is the "kissing spot" on the top of the head.

intelligent and extremely independent, they are seldom aggressive. Any sign of viciousness is a fault.

Head: The skull is slightly rounded with a narrow forehead, barely perceptible stop, and a moderately tapering muzzle. The skull and muzzle should be approximately equal in length. A lozenge or "kiss spot" on forehead is highly desirable, but is not heavily penalized if missing or off center.

Ears: The ears are large and pricked; they may fold back at rest and when gaiting. They are wide at the base, set in a direct line back on the skull from the outer corner of the eyes and gently taper to a point. The ear leather is extremely thin, almost transparent. Surgically altered ears are a fault.

Eyes: The eyes are moderately full and somewhat almond-shaped. The color may be gold in dogs with light gold markings to a black/brown in dogs with darker pigmentation. Completely filled in eye rims are desirable.

Teeth: Missing premolars are correct. Adults with additional missing teeth should not be faulted, as it is part of the hairless factor. Still, good dentition is preferred. (The club is working to improve the dentition in the hairless variety. Until that time, heavy emphasis is not placed on bites, although a scissors or level bite is ideal.)

Nose and Lips: These may be of any color. Fully pigmented is preferred.

Neck: The neck is long and graceful, with good muscle development. Well arched at the head, blending elegantly into the shoulders.

Body: The boning is light, but strong and substantial. The chest is deep and moderately narrow and reaches almost to the elbows. Ribs are well sprung. Shoulders are sloping and well set back. The back is substantial, long, and practically level from the shoulders to the well-muscled, slightly arched loin. Dogs may roach when cold or nervous. The abdomen is well muscled and clearly drawn up, the rump slightly rounded.

Forelegs: The forelegs are straight and long, from the elbow to the knee. The pasterns are slightly rounded and flexible. Weak pasterns are a fault.

Hind legs: The hind legs are long and powerful, moderately angulated. Thighs are broad and muscular. Well-bent stifles. The hocks are moderately low to the ground, clearly defined. Cow hocks are a fault.

Feet: A hare foot is preferred, with webbing between toes. Good strong claws.

Tail: The tail is long and tapering to a point. It will reach past the hipbone when drawn through the legs. Saber tail when moving. A tail carried between the hind legs when moving is a fault.

Skin and color: The skin should be smooth and supple, warm to the touch. A short, soft fuzz on the skull, lower one-third of tail, or low on the hock is the maximum hair allowed.

Skin color is pink or white, with moderate to heavy mottling of any color, or completely one solid color overall. A dog may not be penalized for scratches or scars on the body. Albino is a disqualification.

Gait: Free flowing, smooth, and lively. The forelegs reach well forward, with good drive in the rear. The feet tend to move closer to the centerline when the dog moves at a fast pace. When coursing, the dog moves into a double suspension gait. Viewed from the back, the hind legs are wider than the front. Weaving, crossing, or hackneyed motion with mincing gait is a fault.

In conformation, both varieties compete for one set of points. Open classes are divided by sex, coat and skin color type (spotted or solid).

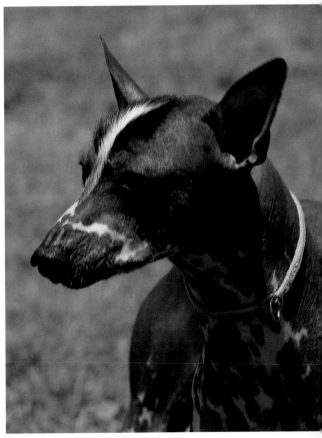

Adult Peruvians tend to be calm and quiet.

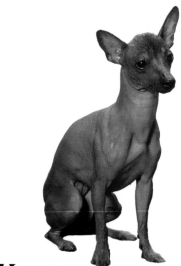

Xoloitzcuintli
(Mexican Hairless)

Pronounce it "show-low-eats-queent-lee." (It can also be spelled "Xoloitzcuintle.") Or, if that's too much of a mouthful, "Mexican Hairless" will suffice. Aficionados call them "Xolos" (pronounced "cholos") for short. This breed is one of the best choices for allergy sufferers, because it produces almost no hair—well, at least the hairless ones produce almost no hair. As is the case with other hairless breeds, both coated and hairless dogs may appear in the same litter. The hairless variety exhibits a total, or almost total, absence of hair. The coated variety is not quite so hypoallergenic; it has a short, flat coat with no thin or bare patches. Xolos are minimal shedders.

This is an extremely ancient breed, dating back over three thousand years, and known to Aztecs, Toltecs, and other Native American groups. The first Xolo owners used them not only as companions and bed-warmers, but also, I am afraid, for food and sacrifice.

Notably calmer than many other small breeds, the Xolo is a restrained animal that barks only under provocation. (Puppies, however, tend to be somewhat noisy.) They are suspicious about strangers and make a good watch dog. The larger sizes can be protective.

Like other hairless breeds, the Xolo must be kept as a house dog, away from sun or cold, and he needs a sweater in the winter and a tee-shirt or sunscreen in the summer. Some Xolos are diggers and escape artists. This is yet another reason not to abandon

The breed's name is a combination of two Aztec words: "Xolotl" the god of monsters and magicians (!) and "itzcuintli" or "dog." There is indeed something magical about the breed.

them unsupervised in the backyard. They are happiest when they are with you.

Some are hard to housetrain, and a few are high-strung. These are sensitive dogs, who react badly to loud noises and harsh correction.

This is a very clean breed—no doggy odor, and no fleas, of course.

Vital Statistics

National Club: Xoloitzcuintle Club USA. Visit them at www.xoloworld.com/xcusa/.

Origin: Mexico, but widespread through South America.

Group: Working (Standard); Non-Sporting (Miniature); Toy (Toy) (AKC.)

Size: The breed comes in three sizes:

Standard: 13 to 22.5 inches (33 to 56 cm).

Miniature: 13 to 18 inches (33 to 76 cm).

Toy: up to 13 inches (33 cm).

Lifespan: 12 to 15 years.

Colors: All colors acceptable. Common colors include black, charcoal, lighter gray, bronze, liver or red. Solid colors are preferred, but spots are acceptable. (Puppies are born pink.)

Grooming: The skin is susceptible to irritation, burns, and scratches. It needs care.

Personality: Calm, alert, thoughtful, cheerful, vivacious, faithful.

Sociability: Good with gentle children, usually good with other animals. However, they need to be socialized early, or may never bond well with the family. A good breeder is very important. Probably not a good choice for very small children. Wary of strangers.

Activity Level: Medium to Low. Daily walks will suffice.

Trainability: High, although they are independent. They are excellent agility and therapy dogs.

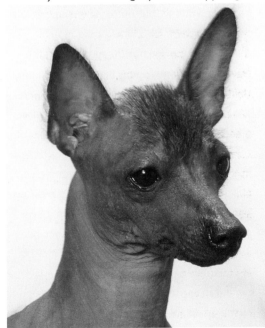

Xolos are sensitive dogs, who react badly to loud noises and harsh correction.

Health Issues: Very few, mostly skin related. Some suffer separation anxiety. Some have drug sensitivities.

Adoption Option: You can find information on Xolo rescue at www.xolorescue.disneyfansites.com/index.html.

Breed Standard in Brief

(From the UKC—hairless variety only)

General Appearance: The Xoloitzcuintli is known for its combination of grace and strength, having the elegance of a sighthound with a terrier's courage and strength.

Head and Skull: The skull is somewhat broad and strong, but not coarse, showing distinctive brow wrinkles when the dog is at attention. The planes of the muzzle and the skull blend smoothly, and the stop is not pronounced. The muzzle is proportionately longer than the skull. Seen in profile, it is wedgelike. The jawline blends smoothly with the base of the muzzle. In profile, it will be slightly curved in its upper line. A strong lower jaw is essential. The lips perfectly cover the teeth and have tight skin. Strong, white teeth meet in a scissors or level bite. Undershot or overshot bites are not acceptable. A complete set of incisors is preferred in the hairless variety, but a lack thereof is not to be penalized. Lack of premolars is acceptable in the hairless variety. The eyes are medium size and almond-shaped. They should not protrude nor be sunken in.

Color ranges from yellow to a very dark brown, with the darker being preferred. Both eyes are to be of the same color. The eyelid pigment will be dark on dark dogs, and self colored or light on self-colored or light dogs. The nose is dark in dark dogs, brown in bronze dogs, and spotted similarly to the rest of the body in spotted dogs. The ears are uncropped, large, and expressive, set rather to the side of the head, and are carried erect when the dog is alert. Ear leather is thin and delicate. Ears not standing erect by 1 year of age are a fault. Cropped ears are a disqualification.

Neck: The neck is proportionately long and slightly arched. It is slender at the point of insertion with the head, widening gradually at the insertion with the body, at the withers.

Forequarters: The shoulder is attached to the upper arm at a 45-degree angle. Shoulder blades are flat and smooth. The point of shoulder angulation should allow for free movement and extended reach, but not so much as to allow the elbows to bow out. The elbows of the forelegs are firm and tight, allowing for reach without elbowing out or toeing in. The forelegs are straight and parallel. They are set well under the body to allow for a long and elegant step. The strong, straight pasterns turn neither in nor out.

Body: The topline is level and firm, with a slight arch over the loin. The croup is rounded and relatively broad. It is neither sunken at the withers nor roached over the loin. The chest is well-developed, the brisket reaching to the point of the elbow. The ribs are well-developed, but not barrel-shaped. Sunken at the withers, roached loin, sunken or roached back is a fault.

Hindquarters: Hindquarter angulation is of proportionate depth to allow for a strong driving rear. A straight or overangulated hock is a serious fault. In the hind legs, the upper thigh is straight and well muscled, but muscular development is not so overdone as to restrict free-flowing movement. The stifle is neither obtuse nor overangulated. When viewed from behind, the rear pasterns, from the hock joint to the feet, are straight. The hocks turn nei-

ther in nor out. Cowhocks are a serious fault.

Feet: The Xolo should have hare feet, with strong, well-arched toes, and smooth, strong pads. Nails are black on dark dogs, although light nails on dogs with little foot pigmentation is acceptable. Hair on the feet of the hairless variety is acceptable. Dewclaws may be removed from both the front and the rear.

Tail: The tail is low-set and fine, reaching to the hock. It may be carried gaily, but not over the back. The hairless variety may have a moderate amount of coarse hair on the lower half of the tail.

Coat and Skin: In mature dogs, the skin is clean, without any wrinkles or dewlap. In young dogs, however, wrinkled skin is still present. In the hairless variety, the presence of a wisp of short, not very dense hair on the forehead, nape, tail, and feet is common. This hair is not soft nor of great length. A very short crest of hair on the top of the skull is acceptable. A total lack of hair in these regions is desirable. Hair on any other areas than the head, nape, tail, and feet is a serious fault:

Color: Any color combination is allowed.

Gait: At a fast trot, movement is free and effortless. As speed increases, the dog will tend to single track, but the legs never incline so far that the feet travel in a single line.

Xolos come in coated and hairless varieties.

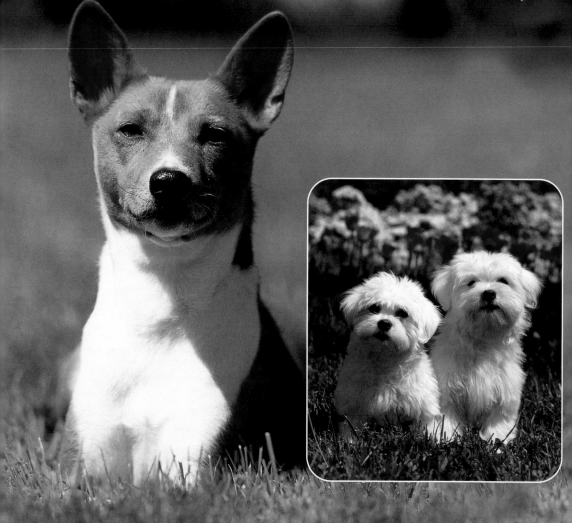

PART 3
SINGLE-COATED AND
LOW-SHEDDING BREEDS

A single-coated dog is less allergenic that one with a double coat, not only because they have less hair, but it is a dog's undercoat that sheds the most. Single-coated dogs have no undercoat to shed. Note: Some terriers and curly-coated breeds, such as the Soft-Coated Wheaten Terrier, Poodle, and Portuguese Water Dog, also have a single coat. Check individual breed listings.

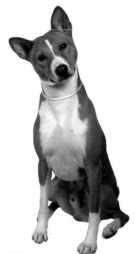

BASENJI

This beautiful African dog is one of the most ancient of all breeds. European explorers originally called them "Congo terriers." The Azande people called them "embwa na bwasenji," which means "dogs from when we were wild."

The hallmark characteristic of Basenji is that they do not bark, at least in the conventional sense. However, they do make yodeling and chortling noises peculiar to the breed. It is a very interesting sound, and one greatly admired by Basenji lovers. (They can also scream.)

This is a very mischievous breed, especially as puppies, who can really wreak havoc! They are also extremely playful and so do well in a house with older, rough-and-tumble children. One of the original names for the breed was *"M'bwa m'kube M'bwa wamwitu,"* which translates into "jumping up and down dog." Indeed. The Basenji will do well in a large apartment if given plenty of time for play and exercise. The Basenji is an excellent climber and, if not given proper attention, can climb his way out of most yards. And, as independent hunting dogs, once gone, they are extremely difficult to get back.

This breed, because of its cleanliness and independence, is often described as "catlike." They are also "primitive." Like wolves, but unlike other dogs, Basenjis come into heat only once a year, usually in the fall. Thus,

The Basenji hunts by both sight and scent.

Grooming: Shirt silky hair that requires minimal care. Minimal to slight shedding. These dogs tend to groom themselves, which does, however, deposit saliva proteins on the coat. They have no doggy odor.

Personality: Cheerful, gentle, proud, rambunctious, affectionate, energetic, independent, curious.

Sociability: Aloof with strangers, good with children, may try to dominate other pets. They tend to bond to one person. They will chase squirrels and rabbits.

Activity Level: Medium to High.

Trainability: High. They should be enrolled in obedience classes early, or they will train you. They are wonderful problem solvers, but less amenable to ordinary dog pursuits like walking at heel.

puppies are usually available only in the late winter.

They have a beautiful coat that, in the chestnut variety, shines like copper. Their movement, too, is beautiful, and has often been compared to that of a racehorse.

Vital Statistics

National Breed Club: The Basenji Club of America. Go to www.basenji.org/.

Origin: Central Africa (Congo region).

Group: Hound (AKC and KC).

Size: 16 to 20 inches (41 to 51 cm); 22 to 25 pounds (10 to 11 kg).

Lifespan: 11 to 13 years.

Colors: Chestnut red (most common), black, tricolor, and brindle. White feet and tail tip. White blaze, legs, and collar optional.

The movement of the Basenji has been compared to that of a racehorse.

Health Issues: Eye problems (coloboma, cataracts, corneal dystrophy), Basenji enteropathy, anemia, hernias, hip dysplasia, thyroid problems, persistent papillary membrane, kidney problems (Fanconi syndrome, found also in people but not in other dog breeds), IPSID (immunoproliferative small intestinal disease, also called malabsorption).

Adoption Option: Basenjis will adjust to a new family very well. For information on Basenji rescue, go to www.basenjirescue.org.

Breed Standard in Brief

(Adapted from the Basenji Club of America)

General Appearance: The Basenji is a small, short-haired hunting dog. It is short backed and lightly built, appearing high on the leg compared to its length. The wrinkled head is proudly carried on a well-arched neck, and the tail is set high and curled. Elegant and graceful, the whole demeanor is one of poise and inquiring alertness. The balanced structure and the smooth musculature enable it to move with ease and agility.

Size, Proportion, Substance: Ideal height for males is 17 inches (43 cm) and females 16 inches (41 cm), measured from ground to point of buttocks. Approximate weight for males 24 pounds (11 kg) and females, 22 pounds (10 kg). Lightly built within this height-to-weight ratio.

Head: The head is proudly carried. The eyes are dark hazel to dark brown, almond-shaped, obliquely set and farseeing. Rims are dark. The ears are erect and slightly hooded, of fine texture and set well forward on top of head. The skull is flat, well-chiseled, and of medium width, tapering toward the eyes. The foreface tapers from eye to muzzle, with a perceptible stop. The muzzle is shorter than the skull, neither coarse nor snipey, but with rounded cushions. Wrinkles appear on the forehead when ears are erect, and are fine and profuse. Side wrinkles are desirable, but should never be exaggerated into dewlaps. Wrinkles are most noticeable in puppies and, because of lack of shadowing, less noticeable in blacks, tricolors, and brindles. The nose is preferably black. The teeth are evenly aligned with a scissors bite.

Neck, Topline, Body: The neck is of good length, well crested and slightly full at the base of throat. It is well set into shoulders. The topline should be level. The body is balanced, with a short back, short coupled and ending in a definite waist. Ribs are moderately sprung, deep to elbows, and oval. Slight forechest is present in front of the point of the shoulder. Chest is of medium width. Tail

Basenjis should be enrolled in obedience classes early, or they will train you.

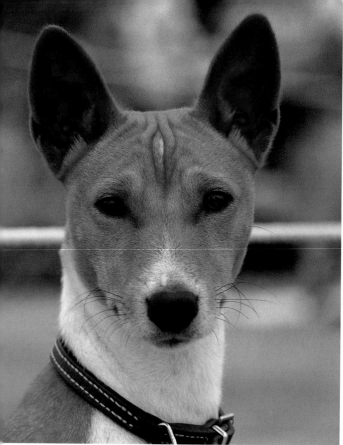

The Basenji is an intelligent, independent, but affectionate and alert breed.

compact with thick pads and well-arched toes. Dewclaws are usually removed.

Hindquarters: Medium width, strong and muscular, the hocks are well let down and turn neither in nor out, with long second thighs and moderately bent stifles. Feet are the same as in front.

Coat and Color: Coat short and fine. Skin very pliant. Colors are chestnut red; pure black; tricolor (pure black and chestnut red); or brindle (black stripes on a background of chestnut red); all with white feet, chest, and tail tip. White legs, blaze, and collar optional. The amount of white should never predominate over the primary color. Color and markings should be rich, clear, and well-defined, with a distinct line of demarcation between the black and red of tricolors and the stripes of brindles.

Gait: Swift, tireless trot. Stride is long, smooth, effortless, and the topline remains level. Coming and going, the straight column of bones from shoulder joint to foot and from hip joint to pad remains unbroken, converging toward the centerline under the body. The faster the trot, the greater the convergence.

Temperament: An intelligent, independent, but affectionate and alert breed. Can be aloof with strangers.

is set high on topline, bends acutely forward, and lies well curled over to either side.

Forequarters: Shoulders are moderately laid back. The shoulder blade and upper arm are of approximately equal length. Elbows are tucked firmly against brisket. Legs are straight with clean fine bone, long forearm, and well-defined sinews. Pasterns are of good length, strong and flexible. Feet are small, oval, and

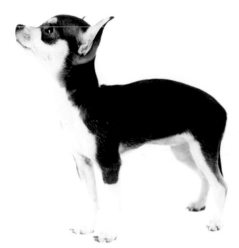

CHIHUAHUA

One of the world's most instantly recognized dogs (as well as the smallest), the Chihuahua is descended from the Techichi, a dog bred by the Toltec people of ancient Mexico. The Techichi was quite a bit larger than today's Chihuahua, though. The ancient Mexicans believed that Chihuahuas guided human souls through the underworld. Chihuahua-like dogs have been found in ancient Egyptian tombs (although it's hard to figure out how they got there from Mexico).

Some arguments exist as to whether the Chihuahua is truly hypoallergenic. People have had extraordinarily different experiences with them.

This intelligent breed lives a very long time, and they excel at obedience and even agility. They make excellent companion dogs. However, the Chihuahua cannot tolerate cold.

Vital Statistics

National Breed Club: Chihuahua Club of America. Visit them at www.chihuahuaclubofamerica.com.

Origin: Central Mexico, antiquity.

Group: Toy (AKC and KC).

Size: 6 to 10 inches (15 to 25 cm); 2 to 6. pounds (1 to 3 kg).

Lifespan: 16 to 18 years.

Colors: Any colors and marking permitted.

Grooming: Chihuahuas come in two types—smooth and long-haired. The smooth variety sheds lightly all year. The long-haired sheds seasonally. The long-haired type requires more grooming than the smooth.

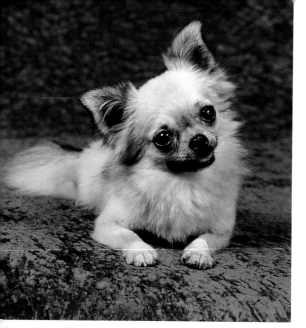

Chihuahuas bond strongly to their owners.

Personality: Alert, loyal, temperamental, courageous, playful. Some can be possessive.

Sociability: Not good with young children, but
fine with gentle older children. They bond
strongly to their owners. Get along well with
other Chihuahuas, less well with other breeds.
This is especially true of the smooth-coated
variety. They need early socialization.

Activity Level: Low to Medium, but does
require exercise.

Trainability: Medium to High.

Health Issues: Heart disease, cancer, dental
problems, hypoglycemia, orthopedic problems
(luxating patella).

Adoption Option: Chihuahua Rescue and
Transport (CRT) is a nonprofit, voluntary

organization dedicated to the rescue, adoption, and the medical care of stray and home-
less Chihuahuas in need, and to help control
the growing overpopulation through spaying
and neutering all dogs in their care. Visit them
at www.chihuahua-rescue.com.

Breed Standard in Brief

(Adapted from the Chihuahua Club of America)

General Appearance: A graceful, alert,
swift-moving little dog with saucy expression,
compact, and with terrier-like qualities of temperament.

Size, Proportion, Substance: A well-balanced little dog not to exceed 6 pounds (3
kg). The body is off-square; hence, slightly
longer when measured from point of shoulder
to point of buttocks, than height at the with-

THE MOLERA

**Many Chihuahuas have a "soft spot"
on the top of the head. This spot, or
fontanel, is called a molera and is the
same as that found in human babies.
The molera may vary in shape and size
when present. Formerly, this molera
was accepted as a mark of purity in the
breed, and it is still mentioned in most
Chihuahua breed standards the world
over. However, many Chihuahua puppies are born without the molera.**

ers. Somewhat shorter bodies are preferred in males. Disqualification: Any dog over 6 pounds (3 kg) in weight.

Head: A well-rounded "apple dome" skull, with or without molera. Expression is saucy. Eyes are full, but not protruding, balanced, set well apart, luminous dark or luminous ruby. (Light eyes in blond or white-colored dogs are permissible.) Ears are large, erect, held more upright when alert, but flaring to the sides at a 45 degree angle when in repose, giving breadth between the ears. Broken down or cropped ears are disqualifications. The muzzle is moderately short, slightly pointed. Cheeks and jaws are lean. The nose is self-colored in blond types, or black. In moles, blues, and chocolates, they are self-colored. In blond types, a pink nose permissible. The bite is level or scissors. An overshot or undershot bite, or any distortion of the bite or jaw, should be penalized as a serious fault.

Neck, Topline, Body: The neck is slightly arched, gracefully sloping into lean shoulders. The topline is level. The ribs are rounded and well sprung (but not too much "barrel-shaped"). The tail is moderately long, carried sickle, either up or out, or in a loop

over the back, with tip just touching the back. (Never tucked between legs.) Cropped tail and bobtail are disqualifications.

Forequarters: The shoulders are lean, sloping into a slightly broadening support

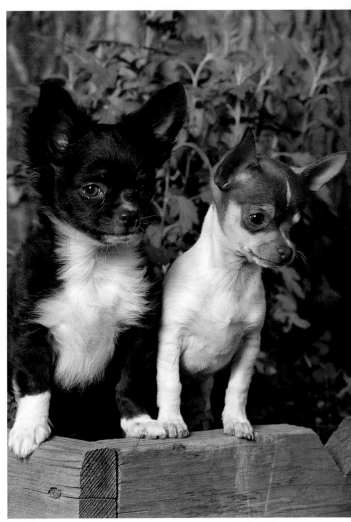

The Chihuahua comes in smooth and long-haired types.

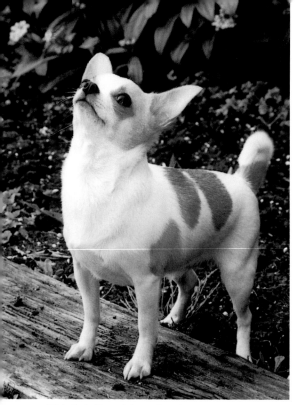

This intelligent breed makes an excellent companion dog.

(Heavier coats with undercoats permissible.) The coat is placed well over body, with a ruff on the neck preferred, and more scanty on head and ears. Hair on tail is preferred furry. In Long Coats, the coat should be of a soft texture, either flat or slightly curly, with undercoat preferred. The ears are fringed. (Heavily fringed ears may be tipped slightly if due to the fringes and not to weak ear leather, never down.) The tail is full and long (as a plume). Feathering on feet and legs, pants on hind legs, and large ruff on the neck is desired and preferred. In Long Coats, a too thin coat that resembles bareness is a disqualification.

Color: Any color, solid, marked, or splashed.

Gait: The Chihuahua should move swiftly with a firm, sturdy action, with good reach in front equal to the drive from the rear. From the rear, the hocks remain parallel to each other, and the foot fall of the rear legs follows directly behind that of the forelegs. The legs, both front and rear, will tend to converge slightly toward a central line of gravity as speed increases. The side view shows good, strong drive in the rear and plenty of reach in the front, with head carried high. The topline should remain firm and the backline level as the dog moves.

Temperament: Alert, with terrier-like qualities.

above straight forelegs that set well under, giving a free play at the elbows. Shoulders should be well up, giving balance and soundness, sloping into a level back. The feet are small and dainty, with toes well split up but not spread, pads cushioned. (Neither the hare nor the cat foot.) Pasterns are fine.

Hindquarters: Muscular, with hocks well apart, neither out nor in, well let down, firm and sturdy. The feet are as in front.

Coat: In the Smooth Coats, the coat should be of soft texture, close, and glossy.

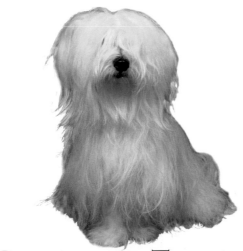

Coton de Tulear

The name is pronounced "coe-TAWN day TULE-ee-r," and means "cotton of Tulear." (Tulear is a port city in Madagascar.) Certainly, the dog has a very cottony coat! This is the Royal Dog of Madagascar. At one time, the Coton was exclusively the dog of Royal Malagasy nobles.

The breed is probably related to the Bichon Frise, although some hunting dog genes were introduced into the lines to give this breed much more stamina. The French colonial rulers of the Madagascar took a fancy to the breed and brought it back to France, where it remains quite popular. Sadly, the breed is nearly extinct in its native land.

These are relatively quiet dogs, not barkers. The Coton is a super companion dog. He loves to run and, not surprisingly, considering his island origin, is also an excellent swimmer.

They are easy to housetrain, gentle, and laid back, getting along quite well with kids and other pets. They love to play and are not as delicate as many of the other smaller breeds. They "stay puppies" throughout their long lives!

Vital Statistics

National Breed Club: **United States of America Coton de Tulear Breed Club. Visit them at www.usactc.org**

Origin: **Madagascar.**

Group: N/A.

Size: 10 to 12 inches (25 to 32 cm); 11 to 15 pounds (5t o 7 kg). A taller variety of Coton is known, but has yet to be described within any standard.

Warning: Because there is yet no generally accepted overarching breed club, many dogs sold as genuine Cotons are not! Your best bet is to talk to a breeder who is a member of the Coton de Tulear Club of America.

Lifespan: 14 to 16 years.

Colors: Usually white. Other colors include white with champagne color patches, black-and-white, and tricolor, (mostly white with champagne patches and a faint, irregular "dusting" of black hairs).

Grooming: The coat is heavy and cotton-like in texture, as his name suggests. Very little shedding and dander, no doggy odor. Soft, wind-blown hair, comparatively easy to groom. The dead hair will come out in the brush, not in your house.

Personality: Lively, loving, loyal, clownish.

Sociability: Most enjoy the company of children.

Activity Level: Medium to High. He does have a lot of endurance and is, in fact, rather hard to tire out.

Trainability: High.

Health Issues: Few health problems.

Adoption Option: UCARE, the United Coton de Tulear Association for Rescue and Education, Inc., a non–club affiliated organization, has since been created to expand the rescue coverage of Cotons. This nonprofit corporation provides rescue, treatment, spaying and neutering, fostering, and re-homing of abused, neglected, ill, stray, surrendered, and unwanted Cotons. Visit them at www.cotonrescue.us.

The Coton de Tulear's coat is heavy and cotton-like in texture, as his name suggests.

Breed Standard in Brief

(Adapted from the Coton de Tulear Club

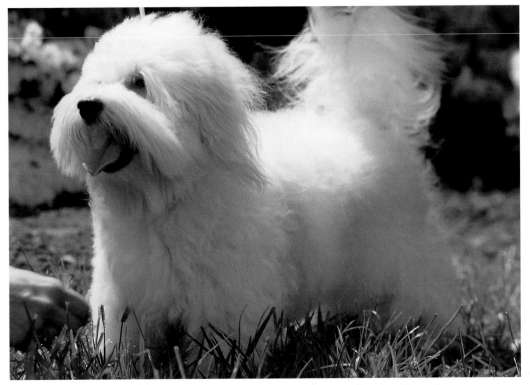

The Coton de Tulear has a lot of endurance and is, in fact, rather hard to tire out.

of America. The AKC does not yet have a standard for the Coton, nor does it register or show Cotons in its regular shows. The Coton de Tulear Club of America does not support AKC membership.)

Head: Skull is somewhat rounded, with proportionate muzzle and slightly accentuated stop. The top-view is triangular. Tape measurement: muzzle to stop, 1.75 to 2.5 inches (4.5 to 6.4 cm); stop to occiput, 4 to 5 inches (10.2 to 12.7 cm); total head length, 6 to 7.25 inches (15.2 to 18.4 cm).

Eyes: Large, dark brown, sparkling, expressive, with dark eye rings. Eye color other than dark brown is fault.

Nose: Black and pronounced.

Lips: Black, finely featured.

Bite: Level or scissors; incisors should touch. Faults: Undershot or overshot bite.

Ears: Dropped, 2.75 to 3.75 inches long (7 to 9.5 cm), covered with long flowing hair approximately 4 to 6.5 inches total length (10.2 to 16.5 cm).

Neck: Rather long, 4 to 6.25 inches (10.2 to

16 cm), strong but gracefully carried, head erect.

Body: Deep chest, tapering slightly to abdomen. Ratio of thoracic to abdominal girth is 1.2–1.4 to 1. Topline (withers to base of tail) is straight to somewhat convex, 12 to 16inches long (30.5 to 40.6 cm). Height at withers is less than 13 inches (33 cm). Body weight is less than 18 pounds (8.2 kg). Little or no sexual dimorphism, but males may appear more muscular than females. Body weight is greater than 18 pounds. (8.2 kg) is a fault.

Legs and Feet: Forelimbs are mostly straight and strong. Hindquarters are slightly angulate with well-muscled thighs. Feet are small with black pads.

Tail: Carried straight or curled over dorsum (no preference), 5.5 to 8.5 inches long (14 to 12.7 cm); covered by flowing hair.

Coat: Long (4 to 6.5 inches; 10.2 to 16.5 cm), dry, "wind-tossed" flowing hair. Texture of cotton, not silky. Prominent beard and moustache. Well-haired limbs, tail, and ears. Eyes may be obscured by hair, which must not be scissored in show dogs, but may be trimmed for pets. Silky or oily hair is fault.

Coloration: Three color varieties are recognized without preference. White: All white, often with champagne (cream-biscuit) highlights on ears and dorsum

Black-and-White: Pure white with prominent black patches on head and body. No restriction on the ratio of white-to-black

Tri-Color: Mostly white and cream, but tinged with beige areas; black hairs dust portions of the ears and sometimes the body and head. Tri-colors are usually heavily marked as neonates and juveniles but, as the adult coat appears, these Cotons may appear almost white.

Grooming: Well-brushed but not scissored. As for any long-haired breed, eyes and ears should be kept clean. The show dog's coat must be natural. Adulteration of the coat (e.g., powdering) is not permissible. Owners are encouraged to ensure that hair is kept trimmed on the feet (between pads and toes), in the ears, and around the anus. Since few Cotons are shown, owners should consider trimming the hair that falls down over the eyes if it is apparent that the Coton's vision is impaired.

Movement: Free, balanced, effortless. Good reach in the forequarters and good drive in the hindquarters. Slight lateral roll at low speed. Legs move straight fore and aft along the line of travel; as speed increases, there is a slight convergence of legs toward the center line.

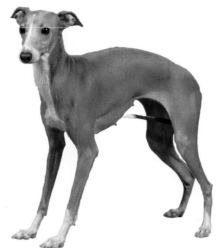

ITALIAN GREYHOUND

This elegant dog is the smallest of the sighthounds. It is believed they originated more than 2,000 years ago in the areas of present-day Greece and Turkey. They are called "Italian" Greyhounds only because they were a fashion craze in 16th century Italy, where miniatures of all kinds were highly regarded. No one is sure now whether this small sighthound was ever really used for hunting or merely bred down from larger Greyhounds to be a pet and companion.

The Italian Greyhound loves to be the center of attention, and adores being inside with his family. They require a great deal of affectionate attention, and can be bored or restless when left alone. Although they are small dogs, they are not "yappers." (They bark like big dogs.) Most tend to be submissive in nature. These make good agility dogs, but have no tolerance for the cold.

Italian Greyhounds were favored by Catherine the Great of Russia, King James I of England, and Queen Victoria, to name a few.

Vital Statistics

National Breed Club: Italian Greyhound Club of America. Visit them at www.italiangrey-hound.org/.

Origin: Middle East.

Group: Toy (AKC) Hound (KC).

Size: 13 to 16 inches; 7 to 14 pounds.

Lifespan: 13 to 16 years. Some have been known to live 18 years.

Colors: Usually black, fawn, red, cream blue,

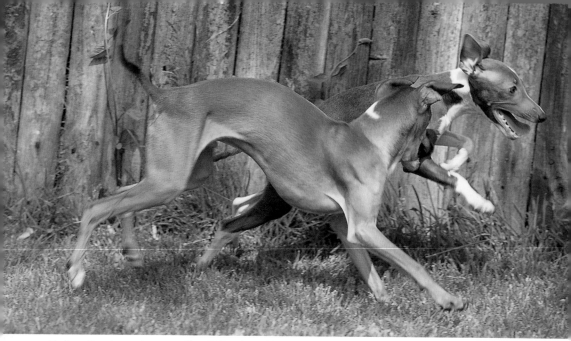

Italian Greyhounds are active little dogs that can do well in organized sports.

with or without broken white. All colors but brindle and black and tan allowed.

Grooming: Short, fine, glossy coat. Minimal grooming. Very little shedding, no doggy odor.

Personality: Gentle, affectionate, calm, alert.

Sociability: This is a peaceful dog. Good with older, gentle children; too fragile for toddlers. Good with other dogs and cats. (Some have to be protected from larger, rambunctious dogs.) He may chase small pets or quarrel with dogs his own size. Some are aloof with strangers. They bond with one person or one family.

Activity Level: Medium to High. Older dogs tend to adapt to the pace of their owners.

Trainability: Medium, with great variation between individuals. Some present housetraining problems because of their dislike of nasty weather.

Health Issues: Tooth and gum problems, progressive retinal atrophy, seizure disorders, Legg-Perthes, hypothyroidism, autoimmune diseases, fractures (in some bloodlines), luxating patella, sensitivity to anesthesia and barbiturates.

Adoption Option: Visit www.italiangreyhound.org/rescue/default.htm for more information.

Breed Standard in Brief

(Adapted from the Italian Greyhound Club of America)

Description: The Italian Greyhound is very

similar to the Greyhound, but much smaller and more slender in all proportions.

Head: Narrow and long, tapering to nose, with a slight suggestion of stop. The skull is rather long, almost flat. The muzzle is long and fine. The nose is dark. A light or partly pigmented nose is a fault. Teeth should meet in a scissors bite. A badly undershot or overshot mouth is a fault. Eyes are dark, bright, medium in size. Very light eyes are a fault. Ears are small, fine in texture; thrown back and folded except when alerted, then carried folded at right angles to the head. Erect or button ears severely penalized.

Neck: Long, slender, and arched.

Body: Of medium length, short-coupled; high at withers, back curved and drooping at hindquarters, the highest point of curve at start of loin, creating a definite tuck-up at flanks.

Shoulders: Long and sloping.

Chest: Deep and narrow.

Forelegs: Long, straight, set well under shoulder; strong pasterns, fine bone.

Hindquarters: Long, well-muscled thigh; hind legs parallel when viewed from behind, hocks well let down, well-bent stifle.

Feet: Harefoot with well-arched toes. Removal of dewclaws optional.

Tail: Slender and tapering to a curved end, long enough to reach the hock; set low, carried low. Ring tail a serious fault, gay tail is a fault.

Coat: Skin fine and supple, hair short, glossy like satin and soft to the touch.

Color: Any color and markings are acceptable except that a dog with brindle markings and a dog with the tan markings normally found on black-and-tan dogs of other breeds must be disqualified.

Action: High stepping and free, front and hind legs to move forward in a straight line. Size: Height at withers, ideally 13 inches to 15 inches (33 to 38 cm).

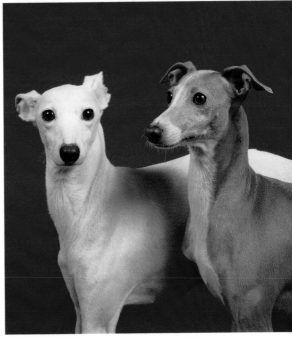

The Italian Greyhound's hair is short, glossy like satin, and soft to the touch.

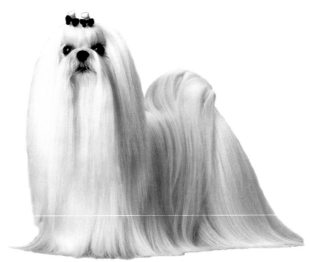

MALTESE

His other names include the Shock Dog, the Comforter, the Spaniel Gentle, and Roman Lady's Lap Dog. The ancient Greeks erected tombs for them. The ancient poet Marcus Valerius Martialis wrote of the Maltese, "More frolicsome that Catulla's sparrow...purer than a dove's kiss...gentler than a maiden...more precious than Indian gems." Indeed— although this description might make more sense if I only knew just how playful Catulla's sparrow really was. (I always thought of sparrows as kind of earnest, hardworking birds; and who was Catulla, anyway?)

Johannes Caius, court physician to Queen Elizabeth I and tireless writer of dogs wrote of the breed, "There is among us another kind of highbred dog...from the island of Melita...very small indeed and chiefly sought after for the pleasure and amusement of women. The smaller the kind, the more pleasing it is; so that they may carry them in their bosoms, in their beds, and in their arms while in their carriages." It not recommended, of course, that hypoallergenic persons do the same. Your little Maltese can sleep quietly in his basket in a separate room.

Many people fall in love with the flowing-coated Maltese they see on TV. However, this showy coat takes an enormous amount of

> The plural of Maltese is Maltese, not Malteses, just as the plural of Japanese is Japanese, not Japaneses.

work and is not practical for most average pet owners—especially allergy sufferers. Show dog owners "wrap" the coat to keep it from matting. Unless you are willing and able to give this dog the grooming required for a long coat, regular clipping at the groomer's will be your best option.

This is a superior apartment dog, although some Maltese tend to be barkers, which does not always suit one's neighbors. These dogs travel well, although they are rather averse to damp weather.

Most Maltese object to dry food, and many need to eat highly nutritious foods three to five times a day to prevent hypoglycemia.

Vital Statistics

National Breed Club: American Maltese Association. Visit them at www.americanmaltese.org.

Origin: Malta or perhaps Melita. (May be originally from Asia.)

Group: Toy (AKC and KC).

Size: 5 to 10 inches (13 to 25 cm); 3 to 7. pounds (1 to 3 kg).

Lifespan: 12 to 16 years.

Colors: Pure white.

Grooming: Hair is long, silky, and single, and

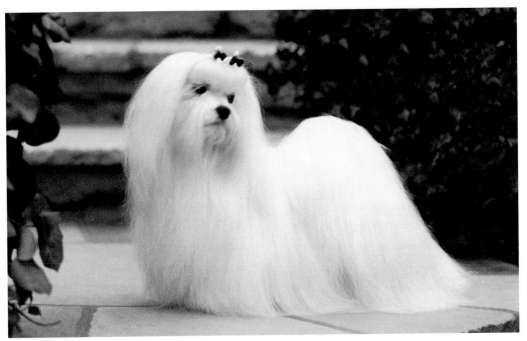

The Maltese has a very high-maintenance coat, but it is minimally shedding.

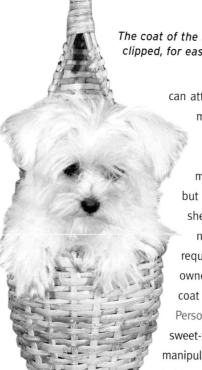

The coat of the Maltese can be clipped, for easier care.

can attain a length of more than 8 inches. It is very high maintenance, but is minimally shedding. Since no clipping is required, dedicated owners can clip the coat themselves.

Personality: Fearless, sweet-tempered, manipulative, loyal, mischievous, outgoing, gentle.

Sociability: Good with older children, good with strangers, although some are reserved. Good with cats, although not always good with other pets. Too fragile for young children, but devoted to his owner.

Activity Level: Low to Medium.

Trainability: Medium to High. Some are hard to housetrain. Puppy kindergarten classes are useful.

Health Issues: Heart problems, luxating patella (slipping kneecaps), white shaker dog syndrome (muscle tremors), tooth problems (retained baby teeth, over crowding), hypo-glycemia in puppies, sensitivity to anesthesia.

Adoption Option: Visit www.americanmaltese.org and click on rescue. The American Maltese Rescue cares for Maltese surrendered by their owners, either privately or through shelters. Maltese that require temporary foster care are kept and loved in preapproved private homes with knowledgeable, caring individuals.

Breed Standard in Brief

(Adapted from the American Maltese Association)

General Appearance: The Maltese is a toy dog covered from head to foot with a mantle of long, silky, white hair. He is affectionate, eager, and sprightly in action, and, despite his size, possessed of the vigor needed for the satisfactory companion.

Head: Of medium length and in proportion to the size of the dog. The skull is slightly rounded on top, the stop moderate. The drop ears are rather low set and heavily feathered with long hair that hangs close to the head. Eyes are set not too far apart; they are very dark and round, their black rims enhancing the gentle yet alert expression. The muzzle is of medium length, fine, and tapered but not snipey. The nose is black. The teeth meet in an even, edge-to-edge bite, or in a scissors bite.

Neck: Sufficient length of neck is desirable as promoting a high carriage of the head.

Body: Compact, the height from the withers to the ground equaling the length from the withers to the root of the tail. Shoulder blades are sloping, the elbows well knit and held close to the body. The back is level, the ribs well sprung. The chest is fairly deep, the loins taut, strong, and just slightly tucked up underneath.

Tail: A long-haired plume is carried gracefully over the back, its tip lying to the side over the quarter.

Legs and Feet: Legs are fine-boned and nicely feathered. Forelegs are straight, their pastern joints well knit and are devoid of appreciable bend. Hind legs are strong and moderately angulated at stifles and hocks. The feet are small and round, with toe pads black. Scraggly hairs on the feet may be trimmed to give a neater appearance.

Coat and Color: The coat is single, that is, without undercoat. It hangs long, flat, and silky over the sides of the body almost, if not quite, to the ground. The long head-hair may be tied up in a topknot or it may be left hanging. Any suggestion of kinkiness, curliness, or woolly texture is objectionable. Color, pure white. Light tan or lemon on the ears is permissible, but not desirable.

Size: Weight under 7 pounds (3 kg), with from 4 to 6 pounds (2 to 3 kg) preferred.

Gait: The Maltese moves with a jaunty, smooth, flowing gait. Viewed from the side, he gives an impression of rapid movement, size considered. In the stride, the forelegs reach straight and free from the shoulders, with elbows close. Hind legs to move in a straight line. Cowhocks or any suggestion of the hind-leg toeing in or out are faults.

Temperament: The Maltese seems to be without fear. He is among the gentlest mannered of all little dogs, yet he is lively and playful as well as vigorous.

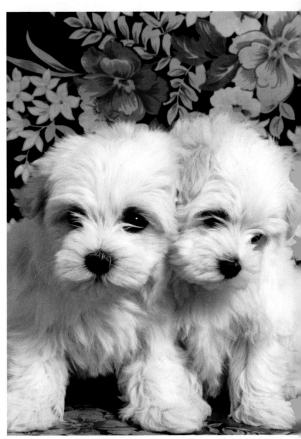

The Maltese is an outgoing and gentle dog.

PART 4
TERRIERS

Most terriers are low shedding and are suitable for people with mild to moderate allergies. Some of the best terriers for the allergic persons include Bedlingtons, Kerry Blues, Soft-Coated Wheatens, and Schnauzers.

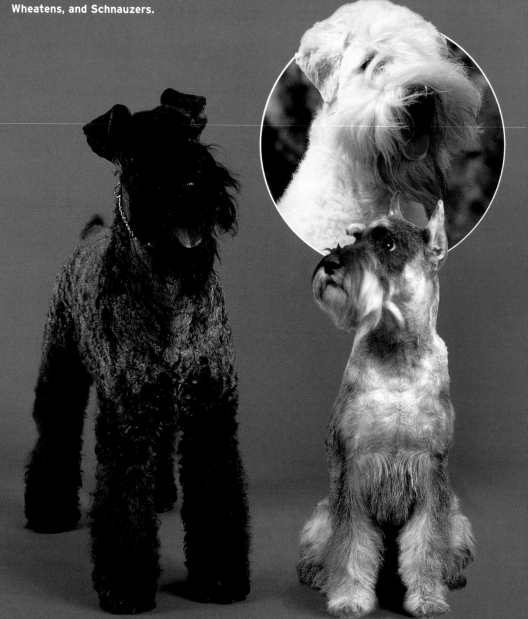

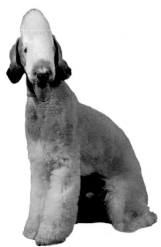

BEDLINGTON TERRIER

The Bedlington Terrier is named after a mining distinct in the north of England. It is believed related to the Dandie Dinmont, Kerry Blue, and Soft-Coated Wheaten Terriers, the latter two breeds also being "hypoallergenic." Some say that both gypsies and poachers made use of the breed to illegally catch game on the estates of the nobility, and the breed was sometimes called the "gypsy dog." It was also known as the Rothbury Terrier or Rothbury Lamb, after Lord Rothbury, the fist "official breeder." In true terrier style, the Bedlington showed his ability to rid residences of rats and other vermin, and so became a valuable addition to the homestead.

An early famous Bedlington was one Ainsley's Piper, whelped in 1825, and who started to hunt at 8 months. It was said he continued to bring down the most ferocious of otters and badgers even in his blind and toothless old age. I don't quite believe this story, but there it is.

The Bedlington Terrier can do well in a large apartment, but some can be barky.

Vital Statistics

National Club: Bedlington Terrier Club of America. Visit them at www.bedlingtonamerica.com.
Origin: Northumberland, UK, 1800s.
Group: Terrier (AKC and KC).
Size: 15 to 17 inches (38 to 43 cm); 17 to 23 pounds (8 to 10 kg).
Lifespan: 15 to 16 years.
Colors: Blue, liver, or sandy. Blue is the most commonly seen color today, although liver was

When bathing the Bedlington Terrier, do not towel dry, as this can cause matting and breakage of the hair. Use a hair dryer set on medium. For precise, step-by-step grooming information for the Bedlington, go to www/clubs.akc.org/btca/grooming/grooming.htm

once preferred. They all mature to a silvery white, peachy white, or peachy brown.

Grooming: Coat is short, linty, wooly, and curly. High maintenance, requires daily brushing and perhaps professional grooming to shape up the coat. Almost no shedding, and does not require stripping, as most other terriers do.

Personality: Companionable, plucky, stubborn, energetic, assertive.

Sociability: Tends to bond with one person. Good with children.

Activity Level: Moderate. While

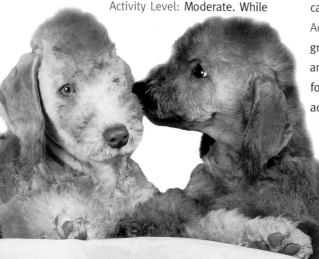

The Bedlington's coat requires daily brushing and profes- sional grooming.

calm in the house, when excited, this breed can run so fast that many believe there is whippet in the background (look at that pro- file!).

Trainability: Low to Medium. The Bedlington does well in conformation, obedience, earth- dog, agility, and is a wonderful therapy dog.

Health Issues: Copper toxicosis (known as Wilson's disease in people, this genetic liver problem first recognized in the breed in 1975), eye disease (progressive retinal atrophy, cataracts, teary eye), kidney failure.

Adoption Option: The Bedlington Rescue pro- gram rescues stray, abandoned, relinquished, and/or impounded Bedlingtons and provides foster care, with the eventual goal being the adoption and placement of the rescued ani- mal. All dogs are spayed or neutered prior to placement. For adoption and rescue information, go to www.bedlingtonamer- ica.com/rescue/index.htm.

Breed Standard in Brief

(Adapted from the Bedlington Terrier Club of America)

General Appearance: A graceful, lithe, well-balanced dog. In repose, the expression is mild and gentle. Aroused, the dog is particularly alert and full of immense energy and courage. Noteworthy for endurance, Bedlingtons also gallop at great speed, as their body outline clearly shows.

Head: Narrow, but deep and rounded. It is shorter in skull and longer in jaw. Covered with a profuse topknot, which is lighter than the color of the body, highest at the crown, and tapering gradually to just back of the nose. There must be no stop, and the unbroken line from crown to nose end reveals a slender head without cheekiness or snipiness. Lips are black in the blue and blue-and-tans and brown in all other solid and bicolors. The eyes are almond-shaped, small, bright, and well sunk. The set is oblique and fairly high on the head. Blues have dark eyes; blue-and-tans, less dark with amber lights; sandies and sandy-and-tans, light hazel; livers and liver-and-tans, slightly darker. Eye rims are black in the blue and blue-and-tans, and brown in all other solid and bicolors. The ears are triangular, with rounded tips, set on low and hanging flat. Point of greatest width is approximately 3 inches (8 cm). The tips reach the corners of the mouth. Thin and velvety in texture, covered with fine hair forming a small silky tassel at the tip. The nose has large, well-defined nostrils. Blues and blue-and-tans have black noses. Livers, liver-and-tans, sandies, and sandy–and-tans have brown

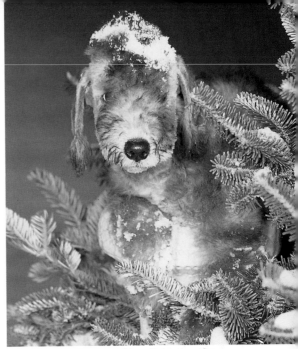

Bedlington's are capable of great endurance.

noses. The jaws are long and tapering. The muzzle is strong and well filled up with bone beneath the eye. Close-fitting lips, no flews. Teeth are large, strong, and white, with a level or scissors bite.

Neck and Shoulders: Long, tapering neck with no throatiness, deep at the base, and rising well up from the shoulders, which are flat and sloping with no excessive musculature. The head is carried high.

Body: Muscular and markedly flexible. The chest is deep. Sides are flat-ribbed and deep through the brisket, which reaches to the elbows. Back has a good natural arch over the loin, creating a definite tuck-up of the under-

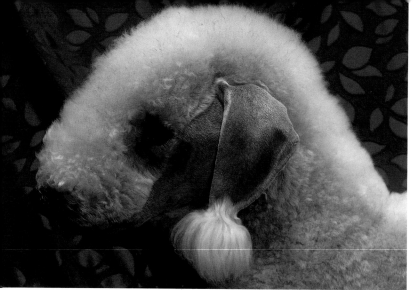

The Bedlington Terrier has a mild and gentle expression.

Tail: Set low, scimitar-shaped, thick at the root, and tapering to a point that reaches the hock. Not carried over the back or tight to the underbody.

Color: Blue, sandy, liver, blue-and-tan, sandy-and-tan, liver-and-tan. In bicolors, the tan markings are found on the legs, chest, under the tail, inside the hindquarters, and over each eye. The topknots of all adults should be lighter than the body color. Patches of darker hair from an injury are not objectionable, because these are only temporary. Darker body pigmentation of all colors is to be encouraged.

Height: The preferred Bedlington Terrier male measures 16 1/2 inches (42 cm) at the withers, the bitch 15 1/2 inches (39 cm). Under 16 inches (41 cm) or over 17 1/2 inches (44 cm) for dogs, and under 15 inches (38 cm) or over 16 1/2 inches (42 cm) for females, are serious faults.

Weight: To be proportionate to height, within the range of 17 to 23 pounds (8 to 10 kg).

Gait: Unique lightness of movement. Springy in the slower paces, not stilted or hackneyed. Must not cross, weave, or paddle.

line. Body slightly greater in length than height. Well-muscled quarters are also fine and graceful.

Legs and Feet: Lithe and muscular. The hind legs are longer than the forelegs, which are straight and wider apart at the chest than at the feet. Slight bend to pasterns, which are long and sloping without weakness. Stifles are well angulated. Hocks are strong and well let down, turning neither in nor out. Long, hare feet with thick, well-closed-up, smooth pads. Dewclaws should be removed.

Coat: A very distinctive mixture of hard and soft hair standing well out from the skin. Crisp to the touch, but not wiry, having a tendency to curl, especially on the head and face. When in show trim, it must not exceed 1 inch on body; hair on legs is slightly longer.

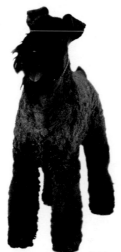

KERRY BLUE TERRIER

The Kerry Blue is an Irish dog developed as all-around working terrier. He was also used for hunting birds and small game on both land and water. One legend says that, since only the nobility were allowed to hunt with the Irish Wolfhound, locals bred the Kerry Blue for poaching purposes. Others say the first Kerry Blue Terrier was either (a) a Russian dog who jumped overboard and swam to shore or (b) a dog who escaped from the Spanish Armada. This dog-from-the-Spanish-Armada story is told of the Skye Terrier and some other breeds as well. The Spanish Armada seems to have had an awful lot of dogs on board, most of whom jumped off.

A Kerry Blue Terrier was named Best in Show in 2003 at the Westminster Kennel Club Show.

The Kerry Blue is an extremely versatile dog who can hunt and retrieve, and has even been used for police work. Some people consider the Irish Blue Terrier the national dog of Ireland, but they'll get a lot of argument from Irish Setter and Irish Wolfhound fanciers, as well as from fans of other breeds. Ireland has no official national dog, although it's said that Irish patriot Michael Collins proposed a proclamation elevating the Kerry Blue Terrier to this role. No records exist, however.

He is friendly, lively, and intelligent, and will do well if given plenty of love. However, he has a true feisty terrier disposition. He also seems to have a sense of humor. The Kerry

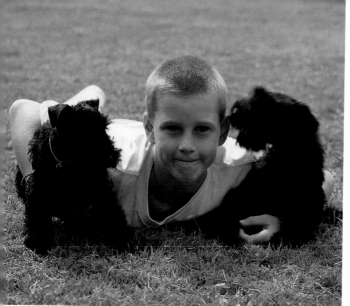

If socialized early, the Kerry Blue Terrier can get along well with older children.

Blue seems to shed dander less than many other breeds (the time for the epidermal "turnover" is once every 3 weeks, much less than most other breeds), but there can be a difference between individuals.

Vital Statistics

National Breed Club: United States Kerry Blue Terrier Club. Visit them at www.uskbtc.com/.

Origin: County Kerry, Ireland.

Group: Terrier (AKC and KC).

Size: 17 to 19 inches (45 to 48 centimeters); 33 to 39 pounds (15 to 17 kilograms).

Lifespan: 13 to 16 years.

Colors: And shade of blue gray.

Grooming: Silkier coat than characteristic of most terriers—can mat overnight. High maintenance, low shedding. The puppy coat is quite different from the adult coat, and a person could be allergic to one kind and not the other.

Personality: Hardworking, affectionate, loyal, adaptable, intense.

Sociability: Very good with well-behaved older children, if socialized early. Pugnacious to strangers and other pets, including other dogs.

Activity Level: Medium to High.

Trainability: Medium, can be stubborn.

Health Issues: Cataracts, bleeding disorders, sebaceous cysts and tumors.

Adoption Option: Many Kerry Blue Terriers are surrendered by owners unprepared for the Kerry Blue high sprits and feisty disposition. USKBTC Rescue is composed of dedicated club members who rescue 30 to 50 Kerries each year. Visit them at www.uskbtc.com/category.php/9.

Breed Standard in Brief

(Adapted from United States Kerry Blue Terrier Club)

General Appearance: The typical Kerry Blue Terrier should be upstanding, well-knit, and in good balance, showing a well-developed and muscular body with definite terrier style and character throughout.

Size, Proportion, Substance: The ideal

adult Kerry should be 18 1/2 inches (47 cm) at the withers for a male, slightly less for a female. The most desirable weight for a fully developed male is from 33 to 40 pounds (15 to 18 kg), females weighing proportionately less. A well-developed and muscular body. Legs moderately long with plenty of bone and muscle.

Head: Long, but not exaggerated, and in good proportion to the rest of the body. Eyes are dark, small, not prominent, well-placed, and with a keen terrier expression. Anything approaching a yellow eye is very undesirable. Ears are V-shaped, small but not out of proportion to the size of the dog, of moderate thickness, carried forward close to the cheeks, with the top of the folded ear slightly above the level of the skull. A "dead," houndlike ear is very undesirable.

The skull is flat, with very slight stop, of but moderate breadth between the ears, and narrowing very slightly to the eyes. Foreface is full and well made up, not falling away appreciably below the eyes but moderately chiseled out to relieve the foreface from wedginess. Jaws are deep, strong, and muscular. Cheeks are clean and level, free from bumpiness. Nose is black, nostrils large and wide. Teeth are strong, white, and either level or scissors. An undershot mouth should be strictly penalized.

Neck, Topline, Body: Neck is clean and moderately long, gradually widening to the shoulders. Back is short, strong and level.

Chest is deep and of but moderate breadth. Ribs are fairly well sprung, deep rather than round. A slight tuck-up. Loin is short and powerful. Tail should be set on high, of moderate length, and carried gaily erect; the straighter the tail the better.

Forequarters: Shoulders are fine, long, and sloping, well laid back and well knit. The elbows hang perpendicularly to the body and working clear of the side in movement. The

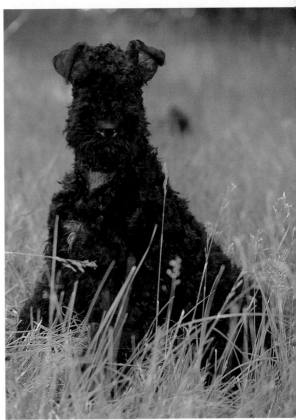

The Kerry Blue has a keen terrier expression.

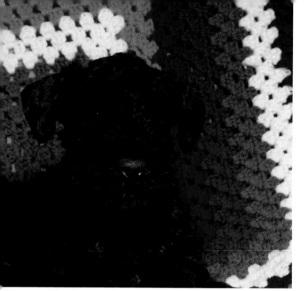

The Kerry Blue has a short, dense, wavy coat.

forelegs should be straight from both front and side view. The pasterns are short, straight, and hardly noticeable. Feet should be strong, compact, fairly round, and moderately small, with good depth of pad free from cracks, the toes arched, turned neither in nor out, with black toenails.

Hindquarters: Strong and muscular with full freedom of action. Thighs are long and powerful, stifles well bent and turned neither in nor out, hocks near the ground and, when viewed from behind, upright and parallel with each other, the dog standing well up on them. Dewclaws on hind legs are a disqualification. Feet are as in front.

Coat: Soft, dense, and wavy. A harsh, wire, or bristle coat should be severely penalized. In show trim, the body should be well covered but tidy, with the head (except for the whiskers) and the ears and cheeks clear.

Color: The correct mature color is any shade of blue gray or gray blue from the deep slate to light blue gray, of a fairly uniform color throughout except that distinctly darker to black parts may appear on the muzzle, head, ears, tail, and feet. Kerry color, in its process of "clearing" from an apparent black at birth to the mature gray blue or blue gray, passes through one or more transitions involving a very dark blue (darker than deep slate), shades or tinges of brown, and mixtures of these, together with a progressive infiltration of the correct mature color. Up to 18 months, such deviations from the correct mature color are permissible without preference and without regard for uniformity. Thereafter, deviation from it to any significant extent must be severely penalized. Solid black is never permissible in the show ring. Up to 18 months, any doubt as to whether a dog is black or a very dark blue should be resolved in favor of the dog, particularly in the case of a puppy. Black on the muzzle, head, ears, tail, and feet is permissible at any age. Solid black is a disqualification.

Gait: Full freedom of action. The elbows hang perpendicularly to the body and work clear of the sides in movement; both forelegs and hind legs should move straight forward when traveling, the stifles turning neither in nor out.

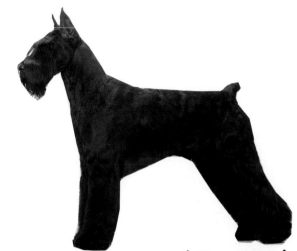

SCHNAUZER (GIANT)

Schnauzers come in three sizes: Standard, Miniature, and Giant. While all are similarly hypoallergenic, these are three separate breeds with three separate standards (unlike Poodles who differ only in size) and of somewhat different temperaments. Therefore, we will consider them separately.

This breed first appeared in Southern Germany, in the nineteenth century, as a cattle herding dog. (Its German name is *Riesenschnauzer.*) At one time, it guarded beer halls and butcher shops in Munich. Many courageous Giant Schnauzers were used in the First World War as combat and messenger dogs, and many of them died of their wounds.

This is a strong, dominant dog who often exhibits guarding behavior of his home and family. These dogs are both versatile and adaptable. They are excellent obedience and tracking dogs. They can show aggression if they are "behind a barrier," but should warm up sufficiently if properly introduced. They have strong territorial instincts. They enjoy being with their families and participating in family activities. The Giant Schnauzer is not well adapted to apartment life.

> Giant Schnauzers insist on being part of the family, but will try to take over unless properly trained.

Vital Statistics

National Breed Club: Giant Schnauzer Club of America. Visit them at www.giantschnauzer-clubofamerica.com/.

Origin: Germany, 1800s.

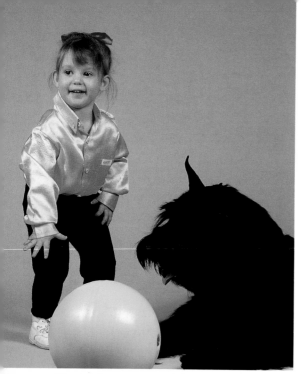

Giant Schnauzers are tolerant and absolutely protective of family children.

Group: Working (AKC and KC).

Size: 23 to 27 inches (58 to 69 cm); 65 to 95 pounds (29 to 43 kg).

Lifespan: 11 to 12 years.

Colors: Black or pepper-and-salt. Some say the pepper-and-salt color is more laid back than the black version.

Grooming: The Giant Schnauzer has a harsh double coat. The outer coat is hard and wiry, the undercoat soft. This is a high-maintenance dog who should be professionally groomed regularly and hand-stripped twice a year.

Personality: Alert, bold, confident, versatile, playful, stubborn, challenging.

Sociability: Tolerant and absolutely protective of family children, but may be too rough for small kids. He may also try to herd them. Tends to bond closely with one person. May be aggressive or dominant to other dogs and reserved around strangers. They can also be predatory with small animals.

Activity Level: Medium to High. Must get exercise or will become restless.

Trainability: Medium to High. However, these dogs must be taught early to accept their owners as their leaders, otherwise they can cause trouble. They are impatient with repetitive tasks.

Health Issues: Hip dysplasia, progressive retinal atrophy.

Adoption Option: The Hertha-Thomas Zagari Giant Schnauzer Rescue is a nonprofit rescue organization within the GSCA. Visit them at www.giantschnauzerclubofamerica.com/rescue/index.html.

Breed Standard in Brief

(Adapted from Giant Schnauzer Club of America)

General Description: The Giant Schnauzer should resemble, as nearly as possible, a larger and more powerful version of the Standard Schnauzer. Robust, strongly built, nearly square in proportion of body length to height at withers, active, sturdy, and well muscled.

Temperament combines spirit and alertness with intelligence and reliability. Composed, watchful, courageous, easily trained, deeply loyal to family, playful, amiable in repose, and a commanding figure when aroused.

Head: Strong, rectangular, and elongated; narrowing slightly from the ears to the eyes, and again from the eyes to the tip of the nose. The total length of the head is about one-half the length of the back (withers to set-on of tail). The top line of the muzzle is parallel to the top line of the skull; there is a slight stop that is accentuated by the eyebrows. The skull is moderately broad between the ears. The top of the skull is flat; the skin unwrinkled. The cheeks are flat, but with well-developed chewing muscles. The muzzle is strong and well-filled under the eyes, both parallel and equal in length to the topskull, and ending in a moderately blunt wedge. The nose is large, black, and full. The lips are tight, and not overlapping, black in color. The bite is scissors and has a full complement of sound white teeth. An overshot or undershot bite is a disqualifying fault. The ears, when cropped, are identical in shape and length with pointed tips. They are in balance with the head and are not exaggerated in length. They are set high on the skull and carried perpendicularly at the inner edges with as little bell as possible along the other edges. When uncropped, the ears are V-shaped button ears of medium length and thickness, set high and carried rather high and close to the head. The eyes are medium size, dark brown, and deep-set. They are oval, with lids fitting tightly. Vision is not impaired nor eyes hidden by too long eyebrows. The neck is

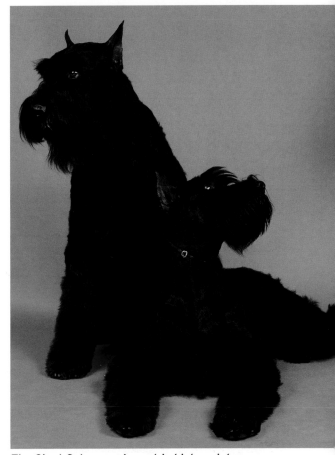

The Giant Schnauzer's coat is high-maintenance— he needs to be professionally groomed regularly and hand-stripped twice a year.

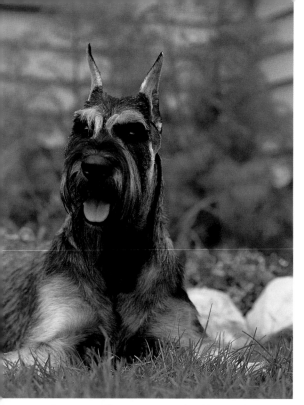

Some say the pepper-and-salt color is more laid back than the black version.

strong and well arched, of moderate length, blending cleanly into the shoulders, and with the skin fitting tightly at the throat.

Body: The body is compact, substantial, short-coupled, and strong. The height at the highest point of the withers equals the body length from breastbone to point of rump. The loin section is well developed, and as short as possible.

Forequarters: The forequarters have flat, somewhat sloping shoulders and high withers. Forelegs are straight and vertical when viewed from all sides, with strong pasterns and good bone. They are separated by a fairly deep brisket. The elbows are set close to the body and point directly backwards. The chest is medium in width, ribs well sprung but with no tendency toward a barrel chest; deep through the brisket. The breastbone is plainly discernible, with strong forechest; the brisket descends at least to the elbows, and ascends gradually toward the rear, with the belly moderately drawn up. The ribs spread gradually from the first rib, to allow space for the elbows to move close to the body. The sloping shoulder blades are strongly muscled, yet flat. They are well laid back so that, from the side, the rounded upper ends are in a nearly vertical line above the elbows. They slope well forward to the point where they join the upper arm, forming as nearly as possible a right angle. Both shoulder blades and upper arm are long, permitting depth of chest at the brisket.

Back: The back is short, straight, strong, and firm.

Tail: The tail is set moderately high and carried high in excitement. It should be docked to the second or not more than the third joint (approximately 1 1/2 to about 3 inches (4 to 8 cm) long at maturity).

Hindquarters: The hindquarters are strongly muscled, in balance with the forequarters; upper thighs are slanting and well bent at the stifles, with the second thighs approximately parallel to an extension of the upper neckline. The legs from the hock joint to the feet are short, perpendicular to the ground while the dog is standing naturally, and from the rear, parallel to each other. The hindquarters do not appear over-built or higher than the shoulders. Croup full and slightly rounded. The feet are well-arched, compact, and catlike, turning neither in nor out, with thick tough pads and dark nails. Dewclaws, if any, on hind legs should be removed; on the forelegs, may be removed.

Gait: The trot is the gait at which movement is judged. Free, balanced, and vigorous, with good reach in the forequarters and good driving power in the hindquarters. Rear and front legs are thrown neither in nor out. When moving at a fast trot, a properly built dog will single-track. Back remains strong, firm, and flat.

Coat: Hard, wiry, very dense; composed of a soft undercoat and a harsh outer coat which, when seen against the grain, stands slightly up off the back, lying neither smooth nor flat. Coarse hair on top of head; harsh beard and eyebrows, the Schnauzer hallmark.

Color: Solid black or pepper-and-salt. In the black dog, a small white spot on the breast is permitted; any other markings are disqualifying faults. In the pepper-and-salt, the outer coat is a combination of banded hairs (white with black and black with white) and some black-and-white hairs, appearing gray from a short distance. Ideally, this is an

intensely pigmented medium gray shade with "peppering" evenly distributed throughout the coat, and a gray undercoat. Every shade of coat has a dark facial mask to emphasize the expression; the color of the mask harmonizes with the shade of the body coat. Eyebrows, whiskers, cheeks, throat, chest, legs, and under tail are lighter in color but include "peppering." Markings are disqualifying faults.

Height: The height at the withers of the male is 25 1/2 to 27 1/2 inches (65 to 70 cm), and of the female, 23 1/2 to 25 1/2 inches (60 to 65 cm), with the mediums being desired. Size alone should never take precedence over type, balance, soundness, and temperament. It should be noted that too-small dogs generally lack the power and too-large dogs, the agility and maneuverability, desired in the working dog.

The judge shall dismiss from the ring any shy or vicious Giant Schnauzer.

Shyness: A dog shall be judged fundamentally shy if, refusing to stand for examination, it repeatedly shrinks away from the judge; if it fears unduly any approach from the rear; if it shies to a marked degree at sudden and unusual noises.

Viciousness: A dog who attacks, or attempts to attack, either the judge or its handler is definitely vicious. An aggressive or belligerent attitude towards other dogs shall not be deemed viciousness.

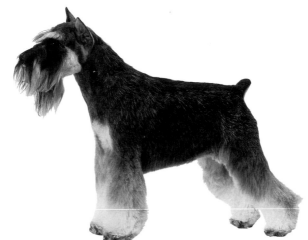

SCHNAUZER (MINIATURE)

The Miniature Schnauzer is derived from the Standard Schnauzer, and he is known in Germany as the *Zwergschnauzer*. The word "schnauzer" means "muzzle" in German. His ancestors may include Miniature Pinschers, Affenpinschers, and Poodles as well as small Standard Schnauzers. The breed was exhibited as a distinct breed as early as 1899.

This is a great companion dog—one who is quick to learn. He is suited for life both in the country and in the city, and is adaptable to many kinds of climate. He is a very affectionate dog who wants to be part of the family at all times and may resent not being allowed to sleep in your bed or bedroom. (You must be strong on this issue, or you'll suffer!) They will bond to the entire family, although they may have a "favorite" within the group. Schnauzers can be barkers. They do well in obedience and agility, and are excellent apartment dogs.

This breed sheds even less than the standard variety.

Vital Statistics

National Club: American Miniature Schnauzer Club. Visit them at www.amsc.us.

Origin: Southern Germany, 1800s.

Group: Terrier (AKC)/Utility (KC).

Size: 12 to 14 inches (30 to 35 cm); 15 to 20 pounds (6 to 8 kg).

Lifespan: 12 to 15 years.

Colors: Salt-and-pepper, black-and-silver, solid black.

Grooming: This is a double-coated breed that has a harsh wiry topcoat and a soft undercoat. The coat requires professional grooming every 5 to 8 weeks for best results. As with most terriers, the coat is best maintained by hand stripping. However, most pet owners opt for merely clipping the dog. (It's cheaper, easier, quicker, and easier on the dog.) This will eliminate the protective topcoat, but the dog will still look neat and trim.

Personality: Friendly, spunky, fearless, energetic, strong-willed.

Sociability: Excellent with people and good with other dogs. Okay with cats. Not good with small pets.

Activity Level: Medium to High.

Trainability: Very high. Probably the most trainable of the terrier breeds.

Health Issues: Eye problems, pancreatitis, pulmonic stenosis, arrhythmia, von Willebrand's disease, skin problems (allergies), diabetes.

Adoption Option: The national club provides a list of resources for those wishing to adopt a Miniature Schnauzer. For more information, go to: www.amsc.us/rescue.html.

Breed Standard in Brief

(Adapted from American Miniature Schnauzer Club)

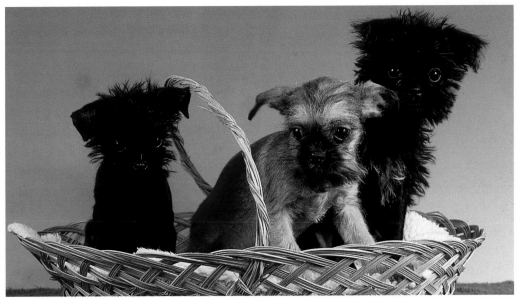

The Miniature Schnauzer is excellent with people and good with other dogs.

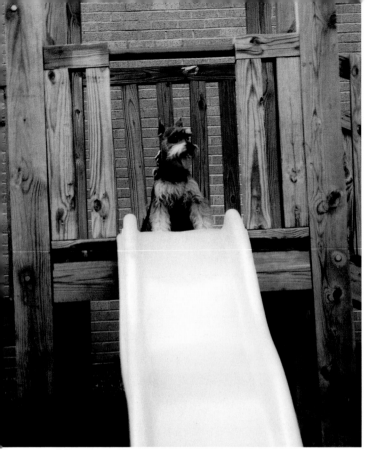

Schnauzers are typically fearless and spunky.

General Appearance: The Miniature Schnauzer is a robust, active dog of terrier type, resembling his larger cousin, the Standard Schnauzer, in general appearance, and of an alert, active disposition. Toyishness, ranginess, or coarseness are faults.

Size, Proportion, Substance: Height ranges from 12 to 14 inches (30 to 36 cm). Animals outside this range are disqualified from the show ring. He is sturdily built, nearly square in

proportion of body length to height, with plenty of bone.

Head: The eyes are small, dark brown, and deep-set. They are oval in appearance and keen in expression. Light or large prominent eyes are faults. When cropped, the ears are identical in shape and length, with pointed tips. They are in balance with the head and not exaggerated in length. They are set high on the skull and carried perpendicularly at the inner edges, with as little bell as possible along the outer edges. When uncropped, the ears are small and V-shaped, folding close to the skull. The head is strong and rectangular, its width diminishing slightly from ears to eyes, and again to the tip of the nose. The forehead is unwrinkled. The topskull is flat and fairly long. The foreface is parallel to the topskull, with a slight stop, and it is at least as long as the topskull. The muzzle is strong in proportion to the skull; it ends in a moderately blunt manner, with thick whiskers, which accentuate the rectangular shape of the head. A coarse or cheeky head is a fault. The teeth meet in a scissors bite. An undershot or overshot jaw or a level bite is fault.

Neck, Topline, Body: The neck is strong

and well arched, blending into the shoulders, and with the skin fitting tightly at the throat. The body is short and deep, with the brisket extending at least to the elbows. Ribs are well sprung and deep, extending well back to a short loin. The underbody does not present a tucked-up appearance at the flank. The backline is straight, declining slightly from the withers to the base of the tail. The overall length from chest to buttocks appears to equal the height at the withers. A chest too broad or shallow in brisket, or a hollow or roach back is a fault. The tail is set high and carried erect. It is docked only long enough to be clearly visible over the backline of the body when the dog is in proper length of coat. A tail set too low is a fault.

Forequarters: The forelegs are straight and parallel when viewed from all sides. They have strong pasterns and good bone. They are separated by a fairly deep brisket. The elbows are close, and the ribs spread gradually from the first rib. Loose elbows are a fault. The sloping shoulders are muscled, yet flat and clean. They are well laid back, so that, from the side, the tips of the shoulder blades are in a nearly vertical line above the elbow. The tips of the blades are placed closely together. They slope forward and downward at an angulation that permits the maximum forward extension of the

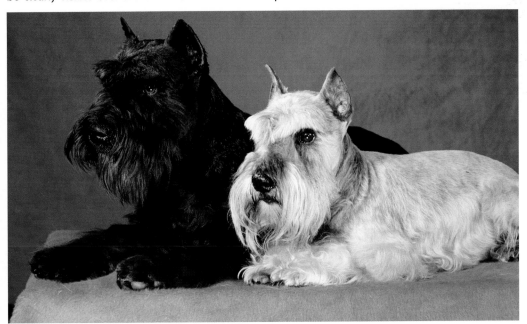

Miniature Schnauzers come in black, salt-and-pepper, and black-and-silver.

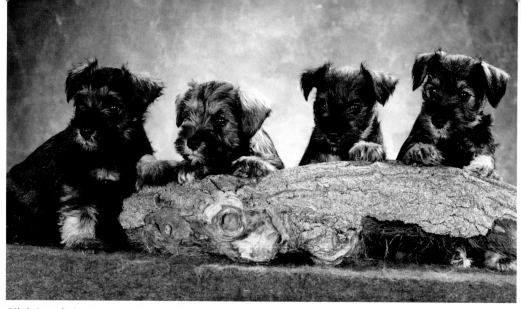

Miniature Schnauzers make excellent apartment dogs.

forelegs, without binding or effort. Both the shoulder blades and upper arms are long. The feet are short and round with thick, black pads. The toes are arched and compact.

Hindquarters: The hindquarters have strong-muscled, slanting thighs. They are well bent at the stifles. There is sufficient angulation so that, in stance, the hocks extend beyond the tail. The hindquarters never appear overbuilt or higher than the shoulders. The rear pasterns are short and, in stance, perpendicular to the ground and, when viewed from the rear, are parallel to each other. Sickle hocks, cow hocks, open hocks, or bowed hindquarters are faults.

Coat: The coat is double, with a hard, wiry, outer coat and close undercoat. The head, neck, ears, chest, tail, and body coat must be plucked for show. When in show condition, the body coat should be of sufficient length to determine texture. Close covering on neck, ears, and skull. Furnishings are fairly thick but not silky. A coat that is too soft or too smooth and slick in appearance is a fault.

Color: The recognized colors are salt-and-pepper, black-and-silver, and solid black. All colors have uniform skin pigmentation; that, is with no white or pink skin patches appearing anywhere on the dog. Salt-and-pepper: The typical salt-and-pepper color of the topcoat results from the combination of black-and-white banded hairs and solid black and white unbanded hairs, with the banded hairs predominating. Acceptable are all shades of salt-

and-pepper, from light to dark mixtures with tan shadings permissible in the banded or unbanded hair of the topcoat. In salt-and-pepper dogs, the salt-and-pepper mixture fades out to light gray or silver white in the eyebrows, whiskers, cheeks, under throat, inside ears, across chest, under tail, leg furnishings, and inside hind legs. It may or may not also fade out on the underbody. However, if so, the lighter underbody hair is not to rise higher on the sides of the body than the front elbows. Black-and-silver: The black-and-silver generally follows the same pattern as the salt-and-pepper. The entire salt-and-pepper section must be black. The black color in the topcoat of the black-and-silver is a true rich color with black undercoat. The stripped portion is free from any fading or brown tinge and the underbody should be dark. Black is the only solid color allowed. Ideally, the black color in the topcoat is a true, rich glossy solid color, with the undercoat being less intense, a soft matting shade of black. This is natural and should not be penalized in any way. The stripped portion is free from any fading or brown tinge. The scissored and clipped areas have lighter shades of black. A small white spot on the chest is permitted, as is an occasional single white hair elsewhere on the body.

Some consider the Schnauzer the most trainable of the terrier breeds.

Solid white colors or white striping, patching, or spotting on the colored areas of the dog, except for the small white spot permitted on the chest of the black, is a disqualification. The body coat color in salt-and-pepper and black-and-silver dogs fades out to light gray or silver white under the throat and across the chest. Between them, there exists a natural body coat color. Any irregular or connecting blaze or white mark in this section is considered a white patch on the body, which is also a disqualification.

Gait: The trot is the gait at which movement is judged. When approaching, the forelegs, with elbows close to the body, move straight forward, neither too close nor too far apart. Going away, the hind legs are straight and travel in the same planes as the forelegs. Viewed from the side, the forelegs have good reach, while the hind legs have strong drive, with good pickup of the hocks. The feet turn neither inward nor outward.

Single tracking, sidegaiting, paddling in front, hackney action, and weak rear action are faults.

Temperament: The typical Miniature Schnauzer is alert and spirited, yet obedient to command. He is friendly, intelligent, and willing to please. He should never be overaggressive or timid.

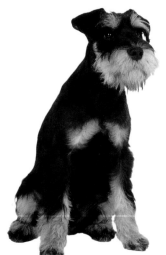

Schnauzer (Standard)

The word Schnauzer means "snout." It is believed the breed originated by crossing black Poodles with the "Wolf Spitz," a breed that doesn't exist anymore (and sounds pretty scary). Apparently some pinschers got involved in the cross-breeding action, too. The Schnauzer's typical salt-and-pepper appearance comes from the Wolf Spitz, while the pinscher contributed the fawn-colored undercoat. The original Schnauzers were used to catch rats, guard yards, and carry dispatches during times of war. They can also make great water dogs, even retrieving in water (that's the Poodle in them). The character of the dog reflects this history: strong, fearless, and protective. This is also dog who can take any weather.

The Standard Schnauzer is the prototype for the other two sizes. They are not known for barking, but when they do bark, it is pretty loud. They participate successfully in agility, herding, and obedience.

Vital Statistics

National Breed Club: Standard Schnauzer Club of America. Visit them at www.standardschnauzer.org/staging/index.html.

Origin: Germany, during the Middle Ages.

Group: Working Group (AKC)/Utility Group (KC).

Size: 17 to 19 inches (43 to 48 cm); 45 pounds (20 kg).

Lifespan: 12 to 15 years.

Colors: Salt-and-pepper; black.

Grooming: Professional grooming. Show dogs require hand-stripping every 4 to 6 months. While most house pets are simply clipped by a pet groomer, this will cause the coat to soft-

The Standard Schnauzer is the prototype for the Miniature and Giant Schnauzer.

en over time (even though the dog will look pretty much the same).

Personality: Alert, reliable, adaptable, affectionate, territorial, challenging.

Sociability: Needs thorough early socialization. When properly socialized, they are excellent guardians for the family children. However, they will not accept any form of teasing. They will protect against perceived enemies.

Activity Level: High, and stay active throughout their lives.

Trainability: High.

Health Issues: Pulmonic stenosis.

Adoption Option: Contact the Standard Schnauzer Club of America at www.standard-schnauzer.org/staging/rescuehome.html.

Breed Standard in Brief

(Adapted from the Standard Schnauzer Club of America)

General Appearance: The Standard Schnauzer is a robust, heavy-set dog, sturdily built with good muscle and plenty of bone; square-built in proportion of body length to height. His rugged build and dense harsh coat are accentuated by the hallmark of the breed, the arched eyebrows and the bristly mustache and whiskers.

Size, Proportion, Substance: The ideal height at the highest point of the shoulder blades is 18 1/2 to 19 1/2 inches (47 to 50 cm) for males and 17 1/2 inches to 18 1/2 inches (44 to 47 cm) for females. Dogs measuring over or under these limits must be faulted in proportion to the extent of the deviation. Dogs measuring more than a 1/2 inch (1 cm) over or under these limits must be disqualified. The height at the highest point of the withers equals the length from breastbone to point of rump.

Head: The head is strong, rectangular, and

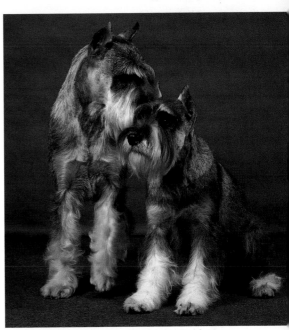

The Standard Schnauzer needs thorough early socialization.

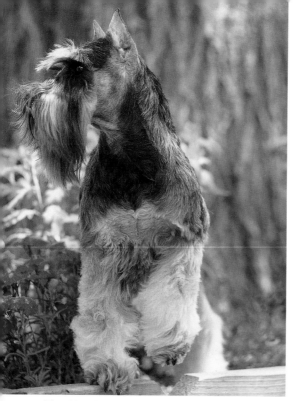

The Standard Schnauzer's coat is tight, hard, wiry, and as thick as possible.

erect when cropped. If uncropped, they are of medium size, V-shaped, and mobile, so that they break at skull level and are carried forward, with the inner edge close to the cheek. Prick or hound ears are a fault. The skull is moderately broad between the ears, with the width of the skull not exceeding two-thirds the length of the skull. The skull must be flat; neither domed nor bumpy; skin unwrinkled. A slight stop is accentuated by the wiry brows. The muzzle is strong and both parallel and equal in length to the topskull; it ends in a moderately blunt wedge, with wiry whiskers accenting the rectangular shape of the head. The topline of the muzzle is parallel with the topline of the skull. The nose is large, black, and full. The lips should be black, tight, and not overlapping. The cheeks show well-developed chewing muscles, but not enough to interfere with the rectangular head form. The teeth are white with a strong, sound, scissors bite. The upper and lower jaws are powerful and neither overshot nor undershot. A level bite is considered undesirable but a lesser fault than an overshot or undershot mouth.

Neck, Topline, Body: The neck is strong, of moderate thickness and length, arched and blending into the shoulders. The skin is tight, fitting closely to the dry throat with no wrinkles or dewlaps. The topline of the back should not be absolutely horizontal, but should have a slightly descending slope from

elongated; narrowing slightly from the ears to the eyes and again to the tip of the nose. The total length of the head is about one-half the length of the back measured from the withers to the set-on of the tail. The expression is alert, highly intelligent, spirited. The eyes are of medium size, dark brown, oval, and turned forward, neither round nor protruding. The brow is arched and wiry, but vision is not impaired nor eyes hidden by too long an eyebrow. The ears set high, evenly shaped with moderate thickness of leather and carried

the first vertebra of the withers to the faintly curved croup and set-on of the tail. The loin is well developed, with the distance from the last rib to the hips as short as possible. The body is compact, strong, short-coupled, and substantial. Too slender or shelly; too bulky or coarse a body is a fault.

The chest is of medium width, with well sprung ribs. The breastbone is plainly discernible. The brisket must descend at least to the elbows and ascend gradually to the rear, with the belly moderately drawn up. Excessive tuck-up is a fault. The croup is full and slightly rounded. Tail set moderately high and carried erect. It is docked to not less than 1 inch (2.5 cm) nor more than 2 inches (5 cm). A squirrel tail is a fault.

Forequarters: The sloping shoulder blades are strongly muscled, yet flat and well laid back. They slope well forward to the point where they join the upper arm, forming as nearly as possible a right angle when seen from the side. The forelegs are straight, vertical, and without any curvature when seen from all sides and are set moderately far apart, with heavy bone; the elbows are set close to the body and point directly to the rear. Dewclaws on the forelegs may be removed. The feet are small and compact, round, with thick pads and strong black nails. The toes are well closed and arched, pointing straight ahead.

Hindquarters: The hindquarters are strongly muscled, in balance with the forequarters, never higher than the shoulders. The thighs are broad with well bent stifles. The second thigh, from knee to hock, is approximately parallel, with an extension of the upper neck line. The legs, from the clearly defined hock joint to the feet, are short and perpendicular to the ground and, when viewed from the rear, are parallel to each other. Dewclaws are generally removed. Feet are as in front.

Coat: The coat is tight, hard, wiry, and as thick as possible, composed of a soft, close undercoat and a harsh outer coat which, when seen against the grain, stands up off the back, lying neither smooth nor flat. The outer coat is trimmed (by plucking) only to accent the body outline. As coat texture is of the greatest importance, a dog may be considered in show coat with back hair measuring from 3/4 to 2 inches (2 to 5 cm) in length. Coat on the ears, head, neck, chest, belly, and under the tail may be closely trimmed to give the desired typical appearance of the breed. On the muzzle and over the eyes, the coat lengthens to form the beard and eyebrows; the hair on the legs is longer than that on the body. These "furnishings" should be of harsh texture and should not be so profuse as to detract from the neat appearance or working capabilities of the dog. Soft, smooth, curly, wavy, or shaggy; too long or too short; too sparse or lacking undercoat; excessive furnishings; lack of fur-

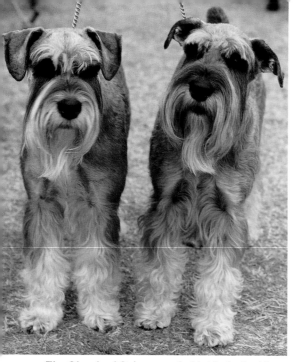

The Standard Schnauzer is highly trainable.

nishings are all faults.

Color: Pepper-and-salt or pure black. The typical pepper-and-salt color of the topcoat results from the combination of black and white hairs, and white hairs banded with black. Acceptable are all shades of pepper-and-salt and dark iron gray to silver gray. Ideally, pepper-and-salt Standard Schnauzers have a gray undercoat, but a tan or fawn undercoat is not to be penalized. It is desirable to have a darker facial mask that harmonizes with the particular shade of coat color. Also, in pepper-and-salt dogs, the pepper-and-salt mixture may fade out to light gray or silver white in the eyebrows, whiskers, cheeks, under throat, across chest, under tail, leg furnishings, under body, and inside legs.

Ideally, the black Standard Schnauzer should be a true, rich color, free from any fading or discoloration or any admixture of gray or tan hairs. The undercoat should also be solid black. However, increased age or continued exposure to the sun may cause a certain amount of fading and burning. A small white smudge on the chest is not a fault. Loss of color as a result of scars from cuts and bites is not a fault.

Gait: Sound, strong, quick, free, true, and level gait with powerful, well-angulated hindquarters that reach out and cover ground. The forelegs reach out in a stride balancing that of the hindquarters. At a trot, the back remains firm and level, without swaying, rolling, or roaching. Gaiting faults include crabbing or weaving; paddling, rolling, swaying; short, choppy, stiff, stilted rear action; front legs that throw out or in (East and West movers); hackney gait, crossing over, or striking in front or rear.

Temperament: The Standard Schnauzer has highly developed senses, intelligence, aptitude for training, fearlessness, endurance, and resistance against weather and illness. His nature combines high-spirited temperament with extreme reliability. Dogs who are shy or appear to be highly nervous should be seriously faulted and dismissed from the ring. Vicious dogs shall be disqualified.

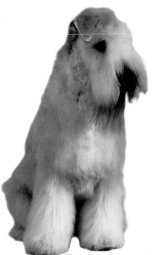

Soft-Coated Wheaten Terrier

The Soft-Coated Wheaten Terrier was bred as an all-purpose farm and family dog in his native Ireland. These are very people-oriented dogs. They also tend to be chasers, and they will run after cars if permitted. They are also jumping dogs and are capable of jumping straight up off the floor to a rather amazing height.

This dog seldom knows fatigue and can handle inclement weather of all kinds, except for excess heat.

The Soft-Coated Wheaten Terrier can be trained to perform many tasks; in fact he has herded sheep as well as performed as a hunting dog.

Vital Statistics

National Breed Club: Soft-Coated Wheaten Terrier Club of America. Visit them at: www.scwtca.org.

Origin: Ireland, 1700s.

Group: Terrier (AKC and KC).

Size: 17 to 19 inches. 30 to 40 pounds.

Lifespan: 12 to14 years.

Colors: Reddish gold to silver.

Grooming: The single, medium, waving, long coat is soft, abundant, and silky. Dissimilar to other terriers. The coat needs to be combed out thoroughly every other day.

Personality: Affectionate, good-natured, merry, steady, friendly. They have an exuberant nature and love to jump.

Sociability: Very sociable in the family. Excellent with older children, too energetic for toddlers. Good with other dogs, not good with cats or small pets.

It is likely that the three long-legged terriers of Ireland—the
Soft Coated Wheaten, the Irish, and the Kerry Blue—all share
a common background

Activity Level: Medium to High. They retain their energy throughout their lives, but can adapt to apartment life if well-exercised.

Trainability: High, but they need intensive work. Heeling is especially difficult for them, and many people have resorted to special harnesses to keep them from pulling. Some individuals attempt to take over the leadership of the family. They are described as "good listeners," who enjoy the sound of your voice.

Health Issues: Kidney problems (protein-losing nephropathy), progressive retinal atrophy, and protein-losing enteropathy (PLE). Addison's disease, renal dysplasia.

Adoption Option: For information about adopting a Soft-Coated Wheaten Terrier, go to www.scwtca.org/rescue.html.

Breed Standard in Brief

(Adapted from Soft-Coated Wheaten Terrier Club of America)

General Appearance: The Soft-Coated Wheaten Terrier is a medium-sized, hardy, well balanced sporting terrier, square in outline. He

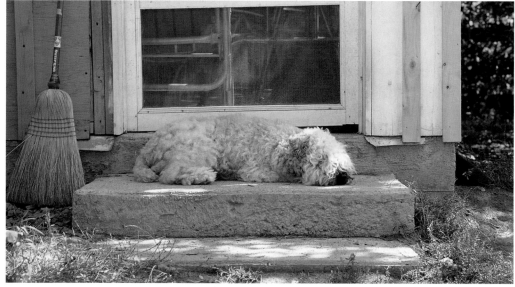

The Soft-Coated Wheaten Terrier is distinguished by his soft, silky, gently waving coat of warm wheaten color.

is distinguished by his soft, silky, gently waving coat of warm wheaten color and his steady disposition. The breed requires moderation both in structure and presentation, and any exaggerations are to be shunned.

Size, Proportion, Substance: A male shall be 18 to 19 inches (46 to 48 cm) at the withers, the ideal being 18 1/2 (47 cm). A female shall be 17 to 18 inches (43 to 46 cm) at the withers, the ideal being 17 1/2 (44 cm). Major faults are dogs under 18 inches (46 cm) or over 19 inches (48 cm); bitches under 17 inches (43 cm) or over 18 inches (46 cm). Square in outline. Hardy, well balanced. Males should weigh 35 to 40 pounds (16 to 18 kg); females 30 to 35 pounds (14 to 16 kg).

Head: Well-balanced, powerful, and in proportion to the body. Rectangular in appearance; moderately long. The eyes are dark reddish brown or brown, medium in size, slightly almond-shaped, and set fairly wide apart. Eye rims are black. Anything approaching a yellow eye is a major fault. Ears are small to medium in size, breaking level with the skull and dropping slightly forward, the inside edge of the ear lying next to the cheek and pointing to the ground rather than to the eye. A hound ear or a high-breaking ear is not typical and should be severely penalized. The skull is flat and clean between ears. Cheekbones are not prominent. A defined stop is present. Muzzle is powerful and strong, well filled below the eyes, with no sug-

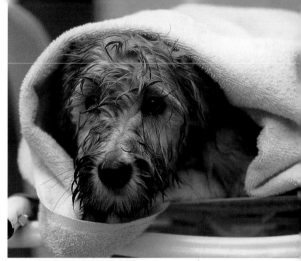

The Wheaten is a happy, steady dog.

gestion of snipiness. Skull and foreface are of equal length. Nose is black and large for size of dog. Any nose color other than solid black is a major fault. Lips are tight and black. Teeth are large, clean, and white; scissors or level bite. An overshot or undershot jaw is a major fault.

Neck, Topline, Body: Neck is medium in length, clean and strong, not throaty. Carried proudly, it gradually widens, blending smoothly into the body. The back is strong and level. The body is compact; relatively short-coupled. The chest is deep. Ribs are well sprung but without roundness. Tail is docked and well set on, carried gaily but never over the back.

Forequarters: Shoulders are well laid back, clean and smooth; well knit. Forelegs are straight and well boned. All dewclaws should be removed. Feet are round and compact, with good depth of pad. Pads are black; nails dark.

Hindquarters: Hind legs are well-developed,

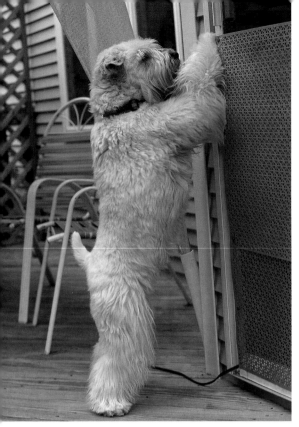

Soft-Coated Wheaten Terriers have an exuberant nature and love to jump.

eyes. Texture is soft and silky, with a gentle wave. In both puppies and adolescents, the mature wavy coat is generally not yet evident. In the adult, woolly or harsh, crisp or cottony, curly or standaway coats are major faults. A straight coat is also objectionable.

Color: Any shade of wheaten. Upon close examination, occasional red, white, or black guard hairs may be found. However, the overall coloring must be clearly wheaten, with no evidence of any other color, except on ears and muzzle, where blue-gray shading is sometimes present. Any color save wheaten is a major fault. Puppies under 1 year may carry deeper coloring and occasional black tipping. The adolescent, under 2 years, is often quite light in color, but must never be white or carry gray other than on ears and muzzle. However, by 2 years of age, the proper wheaten color should be obvious.

Gait: Gait is free, graceful, and lively, with good reach in front and strong drive behind. Front and rear feet turn neither in nor out. Dogs who fail to keep their tails erect when moving should be severely penalized.

Temperament: The Wheaten is a happy, steady dog and shows himself gaily, with an air of self-confidence. He is alert and exhibits interest in his surroundings; exhibits less aggressiveness than is sometimes encouraged in other terriers. Timidity or overaggression is a major fault.

with well-bent stifles turning neither in nor out; hocks are well let down and parallel to each other. All dewclaws should be removed. The presence of dewclaws on the hind legs should be penalized. Feet are round and compact, with good depth of pad. Pads are black; nails dark.

Coat: The coat is a distinguishing characteristic of the breed, which sets the dog apart from all other terriers. An abundant single coat covers the entire body, legs, and head; the coat on the latter falls forward to shade the

Glossary

Agility trials: An organized competition at which dogs negotiate a series of obstacles and jumps in three classes of increasing difficulty (Novice, Open, and Excellent).

Albino: A relatively rare, genetically recessive condition resulting in white hair and pink eyes.

Allergen: A substance, usually a protein, that triggers an allergy.

Allergy: An abnormally high sensitivity to certain substances, such as pollens, dander, foods, or microorganisms. Common symptoms of allergies in humans may include sneezing, itching, and skin rashes.

Almond eyes: An elongated, rather than rounded, eye shape.

American Kennel Club (AKC): The oldest purebred dog registry in the US.

Asthma: A chronic respiratory disease, often arising from allergies, characterized by recurring attacks of labored breathing, chest constriction, breathlessness, and coughing.

Autoimmune disease: A disease resulting from an immune reaction produced by the white blood cells or antibodies acting on the body's own tissues or extracellular proteins.

Bite: The relative position of the upper and lower teeth when the jaws are closed. Bite positions include scissors, level, undershot, or overshot.

Bloat: A sudden dangerous condition in which the stomach fills with gas (and then may twist). Most common in deep-chested dogs and can rapidly lead to death if untreated.

Breed club: An organization of dog fanciers dedicated to the promotion and improvement of a particular breed of dog. Often holds shows or field trials.

Breed rescue: An organization dedicated to finding good homes for unwanted, abused, or abandoned purebred dogs.

Breed standard: A word picture of the perfect dog of any particular breed, drawn up by the breed club.

Brindle: Layering of black hairs in regions of lighter color (usually, fawn, brown, or gray) producing a tiger-striped pattern.

Brisket: The sternum or sometimes the whole thoracic region.

Cao de Agua: Another name for the Portuguese Water Dog.

Cardiomyopathy: A disease of the heart muscle.

Cataract: Opacity of the lens or capsule of the

eye, causing impairment of vision or blindness.

Cat foot: Neat, round foot, with toes held tightly together.

Cheeks: The part of the face below the eyes and beginning at the lips, reaching back to the area in front of the ears.

Chest: The part of the body or trunk that is enclosed by the ribs.

Chiseled: Clean-cut head.

Clip: The method of trimming the coat

Close coupled or short coupled: Comparatively short from the last rib to the beginning of the hindquarters.

Coat: The dog's hair covering. Most breeds have two coats: a harder outer coat and a softer undercoat.

Collar: White ring around the neck.

Conformation: Body type and structure, especially in regard to the breed standard.

Corded: A type of coat that grows in long cord-like strings. Typified by the Komondor and Puli breeds. Poodles will also cord.

Cow-Hocked: Hocks turning in, accompanied by toeing out of rear feet.

Croup: The area of the pelvic girdle, formed by the sacrum and surrounding tissue.

Dander: Tiny scales from the skin, hair, or feathers of an animal that may produce an allergic reaction.

Dentition: Set of teeth. The normal number for an adult dog is 42, for a puppy 28.

Dewclaw: a rudimentary fifth toe high on the inside of the leg.

Dewlap: Loose, pendulous skin under the throat and neck.

Dock: To remove all or part of a dog's tail.

Domed skull: Evenly rounded in topskull (as in the Portuguese Water Dog).

Double coat: A tough protective outer coat plus an undercoat of softer hair for warmth and waterproofing.

Dudley nose: Flesh-colored.

Filled-up face: Smooth facial contours, without excessive muscular development.

Flews: Pendulous upper lip.

Forequarters: The combined front assembly from the shoulder blade to the feet.

Furnishings: The long hair on the extremities (including head and tail) of certain breeds, like Schnauzers.

Gait: Movement pattern, usually judged at the trot in show dogs.

Gay tail: A tail carried above horizontal.

Hare foot: Foot where the two center digits are appreciably longer than the outside and inside toes of the foot.

Hindquarters: Rear assembly of the dog (hips, thighs, hocks, and paws).

Histamine: A physiologically active amine, $C_5H_9N_3$, found in plant and animal tissue and released from mast cells as part of an allergic reaction in humans. It stimulates gastric secretion and causes dilation of capillaries, constriction of bronchial smooth muscle, and lowered blood pressure.

Hock: The joint between the second thigh and the metatarsus; the dog's true heel.

Kennel Club (KC): The major purebred dog registry in the UK.

Layback: The angle of the shoulder blade.

Leather: The flap of the ear.

Let down: Close to the ground, referring to hocks.

Level Bite: When the front teeth of the upper and lower jaws meet exactly edge to edge. Also called even bite, pincer bite, or equal bite.

Loin: The region of the body behind the ribs and in front of the pelvic girdle).

Lure coursing: Organized performance event for sighthounds which consists of chasing an artificial lure over a course.

Luxating patella: A kneecap that tends to slip when the joint is moved.

Molera: Incomplete ossification of the skull, creating a "soft spot," characteristic of many Chihuahuas.

Muzzle: The forward, projecting part of the head.

Obedience trial: An event in which a dog is tested for its ability to obey various commands.

Obliquely set eyes: Eyes with outer corners higher than their inner ones.

Occiput: The back point of the skull.

Oval eye: Egg-shaped eye, characteristics of Poodles and some other breeds.

Overshot: A bite where the incisors of the upper jaw project beyond the incisors of the lower jaw.

Pads: Tough soles of the feet.

Paper foot: Flat foot.

Particolor: Two or more definite, well-broken colors, one of which must be white.

Pastern: The region of the foreleg between the carpus (wrist) and the toes.

Plume: Long fringe of hair on the tail.

Pompon: A rounded tuft of hair left on the end of the tail when the coat is clipped, seen in Poodles.

Progressive Retinal Atrophy (PRA): A progressive, inherited, degeneration of the retina.

Rat tail: A tail where the root is thick and covered with soft curls; hairless at the tip devoid of hair, as in the Irish Water Spaniel.

Ring tail: A tail carried up and around almost in a circle.

Roach back: A convex curvature of the back

Saber tail: A tail that curves upward at the end.

Scissors bite: A bite in which the outer side of the lower incisors touches the inner side of the upper incisors.

Second thigh: The part of the hindquarters from the stifle to the hock, including the tibia and fibula.

Self color: One solid or whole color except for lighter shadings.

Shelly: A shallow, narrow body, lacking the correct amount of bone.

Sickle hocks: Hocks that do not straight on when the hind leg reaches back.

Sighthound: A hound that runs game by sight rather than scent. Also called a gaze-hound.

Single coat: A dog with only one type of coat, usually the outer coat or guard hairs, without the downy undercoat.

Snipey or snippy: A pointed, weak muzzle.

Standoff coat: A long or heavy coat that stands off from the body.

Sternum: A row of eight bones that comprises the floor of the chest.

Stifle: The joint of the hind leg between the thigh and the second thigh. The dog's knee.

Stop: The step up from muzzle to back skull.

Substance: Bone

Throatiness: An excess of loose skin under the throat.

Topknot: A tuft of longer hairs on the head.

Topline: The dog's outline from just behind the withers to the tail set.

Tricolor: A coat of the three colors, usually white, black, and tan.

Tuck-Up: The waist, characterized by markedly shallower body depth at the loin.

Undercoat: Dense, soft, short coat concealed by a longer top coat.

Undershot: A bite where the front teeth of the lower jaw overlap or project beyond the front teeth of the upper jaw when the mouth is closed.

Variety: Division within a breed by size, hair type, or color.

Webbed toes: Toes connected by a skin membrane, seen in many water-retrieving breeds.

Resources

ASSOCIATIONS AND ORGANIZATIONS

Animal Welfare Groups

American Humane Association (AHA)
63 Inverness Drive East
Englewood, CO 80112
Telephone: (303) 792-9900
Fax: 792-5333
www.americanhumane.org

American Society for the Prevention of Cruelty to Animals (ASPCA)
424 E. 92nd Street
New York, NY 10128-6804
Telephone: (212) 876-7700
www.aspca.org

Royal Society for the Prevention of Cruelty to Animals (RSPCA)
Telephone: 0870 3335 999
Fax: 0870 7530 284
www.rspca.org.uk

The Humane Society of the United States (HSUS)
2100 L Street, NW
Washington DC 20037
Telephone: (202) 452-1100
www.hsus.org

Breed Clubs

American Kennel Club (AKC)
5580 Centerview Drive
Raleigh, NC 27606
Telephone: (919) 233-9767
Fax: (919) 233-3627
E-mail: info@akc.org
www.akc.org

Canadian Kennel Club (CKC)
89 Skyway Avenue, Suite 100
Etobicoke, Ontario M9W 6R4
Telephone: (416) 675-5511
Fax: (416) 675-6506
E-mail: information@ckc.ca
www.ckc.ca

Federation Cynologique Internationale (FCI)
Secretariat General de la FCI
Place Albert 1er, 13
B – 6530 Thuin
Belqique
www.fci.be

The Kennel Club
1 Clarges Street
London
W1J 8AB
Telephone: 0870 606 6750
Fax: 0207 518 1058
www.the-kennel-club.org.uk

United Kennel Club (UKC)
100 E. Kilgore Road
Kalamazoo, MI 49002-5584
Telephone: (269) 343-9020
Fax: (269) 343-7037
E-mail: pbickell@ukcdogs.com
www.ukcdogs.com

National Breed Clubs
(alphabetical by breed)

American Hairless Terrier Association
12508 Sam Furr Rd
Huntersville, NC 28078
Telephone: (704) 892-5104
Email: Wudnshu@aol.com
www.ahta.info

The Basenji Club of America
Email: bcoa@basenji.org
www.basenji.org

Bedlington Terrier Club of America
Corresponding Secretary: Mrs. Care Thornton
Email: Corresponding@BedlingtonAmerica.com
www.bedlingtonamerica.com

Bichon Frise Club of America
Corresponding Secretary: Cyndie Adams
Email: leverre@talon.net
www.bichon.org

Chihuahua Club of America
Secretary: Amanda Peterson
www.chihuahuaclubofamerica.com

American Chinese Crested Club
Corresponding Secretary: Marian Blackman
Email: blamm1746@adelphia.net
www.chinesecrestedclub.info

United States of America Coton de Tulear Breed Club
Secretary: Sandi Ramsthal
Email: sandir@hnet.net
www.usactc.org

Giant Schnauzer Club of America
Secretary: Terry Parker
Email: knockknock@volcano.net
www.giantschnauzerclubofamerica.com

Irish Water Spaniel Club of America
Secretary: Debbie Bilardi
Email: cavaniws@linkline
www. clubs.akc.org/iwsc

Italian Greyhound Club of America
Corresponding Secretary: Lilian Barber
Email: iggylil@earthlink.net
www.italiangreyhound.org

United States Kerry Blue Terrier Club
Secretary: Charles Redmon
Email: alainnkbt@msn.com
www.uskbtc.com

Komondor Club of America
Corresponding Secretary: Linda Patrick
Email: cords4me@provide.net
www.clubs.akc.org/kca/

American Maltese Association
Corresponding Secretary: Barbara Miener
2523 N. Starr Street
Tacoma, WA 98403
www.americanmaltese.org

American Miniature Schnauzer Club
Secretary: Ms. Terrie Houck
105 Fite's Creek Road
Mount Holly, NC 28120-1149
Email: secretary@amsc.us
www.amsc.us

Peruvian Inca Orchid Club of America
Secretary: Debby Morris
Email: rarebreedsx2@aol.com
www.willabe.com/index.html

Poodle Club of America
Corresponding Secretary: Ms. Helen Tomb-Taylor
Email: pcasecretary@aol.com
www.poodleclubofamerica.org/usamap.htm

Portuguese Water Dog Club of America
Corresponding Secretary: Catherine Kalb
Email: ckalb@pwdca.org
www.pwdca.org

Puli Club of America
Corresponding Secretary: Michael Rohe
5032 Winton Ridge Lane
Cincinnati, OH 45232
Email: cordonblue1@msn.com
www.puliclub.org

Soft-Coated Wheaten Terrier Club of America
Contact: John Giles
Email: jfgiles@aol.com
www.scwtca.org

Standard Schnauzer Club of America
Secretary: Rise Quay
Email: secretary@standardschnauzer.org
www.standardschnauzer.org/staging/index.html

Xoloitzcuintle Club USA
Corresponding Secretary: Charlene Campbell
P.O. Box 145
Beckwourth, CA 96129
Email: xolomom@webtv.net
www.xoloworld.com/xcusa

VETERINARY AND HEALTH RESOURCES

American Animal Hospital Association (AAHA)
P.O. Box 150899
Denver, CO 80215-0899
Telephone: (303) 986-2800
Fax: (303) 986-1700
E-mail: info@aahanet.org
www.aahanet.org/index.cfm

American College of Veterinary Internal Medicine (ACVIM)
1997 Wadsworth Blvd., Suite A
Lakewood, CO 80214-5293
Telephone: (800) 245-9081
Fax: (303) 231-0880
Email: ACVIM@ACVIM.org
www.acvim.org

American Veterinary Medical Association (AVMA)
1931 North Meacham Road -- Suite 100
Schaumburg, IL 60173
Telephone: (847) 925-8070
Fax: (847) 925-1329
E-mail: avmainfo@avma.org
www.avma.org

ASPCA Animal Poison Control Center
1717 South Philo Road, Suite 36
Urbana, IL 61802
Telephone: (888) 426-4435
www.aspca.org

British Veterinary Association (BVA)
7 Mansfield Street
London
W1G 9NQ
Telephone: 020 7636 6541
Fax: 020 7436 2970
E-mail: bvahq@bva.co.uk
www.bva.co.uk

Canine Eye Registration Foundation (CERF)
VMDB/CERF
1248 Lynn Hall
625 Harrison St.
Purdue University
West Lafayette, IN 47907-2026
Telephone: (765) 494-8179
E-mail: CERF@vmbd.org
www.vmdb.org

Orthopedic Foundation for Animals (OFA)
2300 NE Nifong Blvd
Columbus, Missouri 65201-3856
Telephone: (573) 442-0418
Fax: (573) 875-5073
Email: ofa@offa.org
www.offa.org

MISCELLANEOUS

Association of Pet Dog Trainers (APDT)
150 Executive Center Drive Box 35
Greenville, SC 29615
Telephone: (800) PET-DOGS
Fax: (864) 331-0767
E-mail: information@apdt.com
www.apdt.com

Delta Society
875 124th Ave NE, Suite 101
Bellevue, WA 98005
Telephone: (425) 226-7357
Fax: (425) 235-1076
E-mail: info@deltasociety.org
www.deltasociety.org

Therapy Dogs International (TDI)
88 Bartley Road
Flanders, NJ 07836
Telephone: (973) 252-9800
Fax: (973) 252-7171
E-mail: tdi@gti.net
www.tdi-dog.org

PUBLICATIONS

AKC Family Dog
American Kennel Club
260 Madison Avenue
New York, NY 10016
Telephone: (800) 490-5675
E-mail: familydog@akc.org
www.akc.org/pubs/familydog

AKC Gazette
American Kennel Club
260 Madison Avenue
New York, NY 10016
Telephone: (800) 533-7323
E-mail: gazette@akc.org
www.akc.org/pubs/gazette

Dog & Kennel
Pet Publishing, Inc.
7-L Dundas Circle
Greensboro, NC 27407
Telephone: (336) 292-4272
Fax: (336) 292-4272
E-mail: info@petpublishing.com
www.dogandkennel.com

Dog Fancy
Subscription Department
P.O. Box 53264
Boulder, CO 80322-3264
Telephone: (800) 365-4421
E-mail: barkback@dogfancy.com
www.dogfancy.com

Dogs Monthly
Ascot House
High Street, Ascot,
Berkshire SL5 7JG
United Kingdom
Telephone: 0870 730 8433
Fax: 0870 730 8431
E-mail: admin@rtc-associates.freeserve.co.uk
www.corsini.co.uk/dogsmonthly

WEBSITES

Allergy Related

American College of Allergy, Asthma, and Immunology (ACAAI)
www.acaai.org

National Institute of Environmental Health Sciences (NIEHS)
www.niehs.nih.gov/oc/news/dogcata.htm

Rescue and Adoption
(alphabetical by breed)

American Hairless Terrier Rescue
www.ahta.info/rtrescue.html

Basenji Rescue and Transport
www.basenjirescue.org

Bedlington Rescue
www.bedlingtonamerica.com/rescue/index.htm

US Bichon Frise Rescue Effort
www.bichon.org/usrescueeffort.htm

Chihuahua Rescue & Transport
www.chihuahua-rescue.com

Crest-Care, Inc. [Chinese Crested Rescue]
www.crest-care.com

United Coton de Tulear Association for Rescue and Education
www.cotonrescue.us

The Hertha-Thomas Zagari Giant Schnauzer Rescue
www.giantschnauzerclubofamerica.com/rescue/index.htm

Irish Water Spaniel Rescue
www.clubs.akc.org/iwsc/Rescue/contacts.htm

Italian Greyhound Club of America Rescue
www.italiangreyhound.org/rescue/default.htm

Kerry Blue Terrier Rescue
www.uskbtc.com/category.php/9.

Komondor Club of America Rescue
www.clubs.akc.org/kca/kca.htm

Maltese Rescue
www.americanmaltese.org

Miniature Schnauzer Rescue
www.amsc.us/rescue.html

Portuguese Water Dog Club of America Rescue
www.pwdca.org/rescue.html

Poodle Club of America National Rescue
www.poodleclubofamerica.org

Puli Club of America Rescue
www.puliclub.org/PCARescue.htm

Soft-Coated Wheaten Terrier Rescue
www.scwtca.org/rescue.html

Standard Schnauzer Club of America Rescue
www.standardschnauzer.org/staging/rescue-home.html

Xolo Rescue
www.xolorescue.disneyfansites.com/index.html

Index

A

access restriction of dogs, 34–35
Accolate, 21
Afghan Hounds, 44
age and allergies, 8, 36–37
air conditioning, 26
air filtration and air cleaners, 25–26
Alaskan Malamute, 14, 15
Albert Einstein School of Medicine, 47
Allerca, 46–47
allergen immunotherapy, 17–19
allergen neutralizing products, 35
allergens, 5–6
allergies defined, 8–9
allergist selection, 8
Allergy Relief Center, 30
allergy sufferers, numbers of, in U.S., 5
Allerpet, 28, 36
Allerpet/D and /C, 35
Allersearch ADS Anti-Allergen Dust Spray, 29
Alocril, 21
American College of Allergy, Asthma, and Immunology (ACAAI), 18
American Hairless Terrier, 41, 81–85, **81, 82, 84**
Amitraz, 33
anagen phase of hair growth, 15
anaphylaxis, 11
animal allergies, 5, 13
anti-dander products, 28
antihistamine treatment, 19–21
anti-IgE (rhuMAb–E25) in, 22, 23
Astemizole (Hismanal), 20
asthma and allergies, 5, 7
    treatments for, 21
atopic allergy, 10
Atrovent, 21
Austin Air HEPA Air Cleaners, 26
Azatadine, 20

B

bacterial skin infections on dogs, 33
Basenji, 41, 99–102, **98, 99, 101, 102**
basophils and immune function, 9
Basset Hounds, 44
bathing your dog, 30, **30**
Bearded Collies, 14, 15
bedding and allergens, 23, 36
Bedlington Terrier, 41, 119–122, **119, 120, 121, 122**
bedroom and dogs, 34
Benadryl, 20

B (continued)

Bichon Frise, 41, 51–56, **53, 55, 56**
Bio Spot, 33
Bionair Air Cleaners, 26
blood tests for allergy, 12–13
Blueair air cleaner/filter, 26
bradykinin, 10
Brodie, Simon, 46–47
brompheniramine, 20
brushing your dog, 30–31

C

CARE 2000 air cleaner/filter, 26
carpeting, 23–24
cars and allergens, 28
cat allergens, 6, 15, 46–47
catagen phase of hair growth, 15
Cetirizine, 20
Chihuahua, 41, **42**, 103–106, **103,104, 105, 106**
children and allergies, preventing, 36–37
Chinese Crested, 41, 86–89, **86, 87, 88, 89**
Chinese Shar-Peis, 44
chlorpheniramine, 20
Chlor–Trimeton, 20
Claritin, 20
Clemastine, 20
clothing for dogs, 29
Cocker Spaniel, 40, **43**, 44
controlling allergies, 6
corded-coat breeds, 50–79
corticosteroids for allergy treatment, 21
Coton de Tulear, 41, 107–110, **107, 108, 109**
Cromolyn, 21
curly-coated breeds, 41, 42, 47, 50–79
curtains, 24–25
Cyprohexadine, 20

D

Dachshund, **43**, 44
dander, 5–6, 13
Defend, 33
Delorghi air cleaner/filter, 26
demodectic mange, 33
designer dogs, 39–40, 47
Dexbrompheniramine, 20
dexchlorpheniramine, 20
diet (dog) and allergen production, 31–32
diphenhydramine, 19, 20
Doberman Pinschers, 44
dog bedding hygiene, 36
dog health vs. allergen production, 29–34

E

epinephrine, 19
eye drops for allergy treatment, 21
eye inflammation, 14

F

fatty acids vs. allergen production, 31–32
Fel-d cat allergen, 47
finding the cause of allergy, 12–13
finding the right dog, 45–46
fipronil, 32, 33
flea control, 32–33
Frontline, 33
fungal skin infections on dogs, 33
furniture, 24–25

G

genetic engineering animals, 46–47
German Shepherd, **43**
granulocytes and immune function, 9–10

H

hair and allergy, 15
hairless breeds, 41, 42, 47, 80–97
hand washing and allergy prevention, 26
HEPA filters, 25, 29
histamine, 10–11, 12
    antihistamine treatment for, 19–21
histamine blockers, 19
Honeywell Air Cleaner, 26
hormonal disease in dogs, 34
housecleaning, 29
household allergen presence, 7–8
humidity and allergy, 27
hypoallergenic breeds, 39–47
hypothyroidism in dogs, 34

I

imidacloprid, 32, 33
immune system and allergy, 8–9, 8
immunoglobulin E (IgE), 9–11
immunotherapy, 17–19
insect growth regulators (IGRs), 32
IQAir air cleaner/filter, 26
Irish Setters, 44
Irish Water Spaniel, 41, 57–60, **57, 58, 60**
Italian Greyhound, 41, **42**, 111–113, **111, 112, 113**

J

Job-Buckley syndrome, 11

K

K9 Advantix, 33
Kerry Blue Terrier, 41, 123–126, **123, 124, 125, 126**
Komondor, 41, 42, 61–65, **61, 63, 64**

L

Labraddoodle, 39–40, 47
Labrador, 39, 47
leukotriene modifiers, 21
Lightning Air air cleaner/filter, 26
living with your dog and dog allergy, 6–7
Loratadine, 20
low-shedding breeds, 41, 98–117
lufenuron, 33

M

Maltese, 40, 41, 114–117, **114, 115, 116, 117**
Maltipoo, 40, **41**
mange, 33
Marshall, Gailen, 47
mast cells and immune function, 9
Medical College of Georgia, 37
Methdilazine, 20
methoprene, 33
Mexican Hairless, 94–97, **94, 95, 97**
mite control, 32–33
molera, 104
Mrs. Allen's Shed-Stop, 32

N

nasal sprays, 21–22
NasalCrom, 21
Nasonex, 21
National Institute for Environmental Health Sciences
(NIEHS), 7, 8
Nature's Miracle, 35–36

O

omalizumab (Xolair), 22
Omega 3 and 6 fatty acids vs. allergen production,
31–32
Outright Allergy Relief, 36
Ownby, Dennis R., 37

P

Panasonic air cleaner/filter, 26
parasite control, 32–33
Patanol, 21
perennial allergic rhinitis, 14, 15
permethrin, 32, 33
Peruvian Inca Orchid/Peruvian Hairless, 41, 90–93, **90,
91, 92, 93**
Petal Cleanse/D, 36
pollen allergies, 27–28
Poodle, 39, 40, 41, 47, 65–70, **65, 67, 68, 69**
Portuguese Water Dog, 41, 71–75, **71, 72, 73, 74, 75**
prescription vs. over-the-counter medications, 20
Preventic, 33
Promethazine, 20
prostaglandins, 10
proteins that trigger allergies. *See* allergens

Puli, 41, 42, 76–79, **76**, **77**, **78**, **79**
pyrethrin, 32
Pyrilamine, 20
pyriproxfen, 33
pyrethrin, 33

R
radioallergosorbent (RAST) assay, 13
"rebound effect", 21
receptor cells and immune response, 10
rescue organizations, 45
Revolution, 33
rhuMAb–E25, 22, 23
Rosenstreich, David, 47
runny nose, 14

S
saliva and allergens, 6, 44
sarcoptic mange, 33
Schnauzer, 41
Schnauzer, Giant, 31, 127–131, **127**, **128**, **129**, **130**
Schnauzer, Miniature, 41, 132–137, **132**, **133**, **134**, **135**, **136**
Schnauzer, Standard, 41, 138–142, **138**, **139**, **140**, **142**
scurf, 12
seasonal allergies, 27–28
selamectin, 32
Seldane–D, 20
severe allergic reaction, 11
shedding and allergy, 15, 32, 42
shots in allergy treatment, 17–19
Siberian Husky, **14**, 15
single-coated breeds, 41, 98–117
Singulair, 21
sinus problems and allergy, 14, 15
skin care for dogs, vs. allergen production, 29–30
skin tests for allergies, 13
small breeds, 43–44
smoking and allergies in children, 37
sneezing, 14
Soft-Coated Wheaten Terrier, 41, 143–146, **143**, **144**, **145**, **146**
Springer Spaniels, 44
substance P, 10
Surround Air air cleaner/filter, 26
symptoms of allergy, 5, 10, 13, 14

T
Taskmaster air cleaner/filter, 26
Tavist, 20
Terfenadine, 20
terrier-type breeds, 41, 42, 118–146
tick control, 32–33
topical allergen neutralizing products, 35
toys and dog bedding hygiene, 36

treating and managing allergies, 17–37
    access restriction of dogs in, 34–35
    air filtration and air cleaners in, 25–26
    anti-dander products in, 28
    antihistamine tablets in, 20
    antihistamine treatment in, 19–21
    anti–IgE (rhuMAb–E25) in, 22, 23
    asthma and, 21
    car cleaning and, 28
    corticosteroids in, 21
    dog health care in, 29–34
    eye drops in, 21
    home hygiene and, 23–24
    housecleaning and, 29
    humidity control in, 27
    immunotherapy (shots) in, 17–19
    leukotriene modifiers in, 21
    nasal sprays in, 21–22
    omalizumab (Xolair) in, 22
    prescription vs. over-the-counter medications in, 20
    "rebound effect" and, 21
    side effects of, 20–21
    topical allergen neutralizing products in, 35
    toys and dog bedding hygiene in, 36
    vacuuming in, 28–29, **29**
    ventilation control in, 27–28
Trimeprazine, 20
Tripelennamine, 20
Triprolidine, 20

U
University of Mississippi Medical Center, 47
upholstered furniture, 24
urine and allergens, 6, 13

V
vacuuming vs. allergy, 28–29, **29**
Vent-Pro Heating Vent Filters, 26
ventilation and allergy, 27–28

W
West Highland White Terrier, **43**, 44
wire-haired breeds, 42, 47

X
Xolair, 22
Xoloitzcuintli (Mexican Hairless), 41, 94–97, **94**, **95**, **97**

Z
Zaditor, 21
Zileuton, 21
Zyflo, 21

ABOUT THE AUTHOR

DIANE MORGAN is an award-winning writer who is the author of many books, including *Good Dogkeeping, The Simple Guide to Choosing a Dog,* and *Feeding Your Dog for Life.* She is an ardent supporter of canine res-cue and a charter member and Treasurer of Basset Hound Rescue of Old Dominion. She is a college pro-fessor of philosophy and literature and resides in Williamsport, Maryland with five dogs, two humans, and an uncounted number of goldfish.

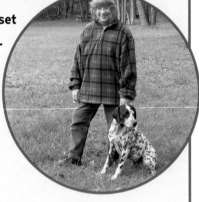

DEDICATION

For John and Helen Seldon in honor of their devotion to Basset Hound Rescue.

ACKNOWLEDGEMENT

Thanks to Dominique DeVito for thinking of me for this project, and especially to Heather Russell-Revesz for her expert editing, patience, and amazing ability to turn a manuscript into a book.

PHOTO CREDITS

Photos on pages 4, 6, 9, 11, 12, 16, 20, 22, 23, 24, 25, 26, 27, 28, 29 (top), 35 courtesy of Lexiann Grant.

Photos on pages 29 (bottom), 41 courtesy of Tilly Grassa.

Photo on page 39 courtesy of Mary Bloom.

Photo on page 81 courtesy of Kristiina MacGregor.

Photos on page 82, 84 courtesy of Therese Murphy.

All other photos courtesy of Isabelle Francais.